WHAT SHE WANTS

WHAT
SHE
WANTS:

A MAN'S
GUIDE TO
WOMEN

CURTIS PESMEN

BALLANTINE BOOKS / NEW YORK

For Mom, Dad, and for Beth

This book is not intended to treat, diagnose, or prescribe. If you or anyone
else have a serious health problem, we suggest you consult a professional
health worker.

Many names of the interviewees in this book have been changed to protect
their privacy.

Library of Congress Catalog Card Number: 91-092156
ISBN: 0-345-36653-0

Cover design by Susan Grube
Cover photograph by Wendi Schneider
Text design by Beth Toudreau Design / Mary A. Wirth

Manufactured in the United States of America
First Ballantine Books Edition: October 1992
10 9 8 7 6

CONTENTS

I didn't know it at the time, but my roommates and I stumbled onto the idea for this book ten years before it was written. There were three of us: Todd, Geoff, and I, Midwesterners just out of college, who in 1980 were living in a fifth-floor walkup on the fringes of Greenwich Village. We had moved to New York City to begin careers in the creative arts and we were taking our first steps into these worlds haphazardly. The same could be said, I suppose, about the ways in which we entered into our first relationships with women.

One night around midnight we got to talking about sex and women's bodies. In a way it was typical guy-talk for men in their early twenties, except that there was a woman in the room, a girlfriend of Todd's. And at one point she began to give us a kind of lecture. One of us had confessed he had trouble figuring women out "down there," so in service to us all (as well as to her gender) she opened a spiral-bound notebook and drew a circle. Then she drew three smaller circles in a vertical row inside the original one. They added up to a rudimentary sketch of female reproductive anatomy.

"*This* is where you put 'it' in," she said, pointing to the vaginal opening on the page, the largest of the three smaller circles. "And this is where we go to the bathroom," pointing to the one just above. "Sex [and petting] hurts us sometimes because they're so close. And it's also why we get so many damn infections." We hadn't even got to the pleasure part of things yet, the clitoris, and what occurred to me was startling: If we three college-educated men living in the most sophisticated city in the world needed help like this when it came to figuring out the raw basics of women's bodies, what about other men? Couldn't at least a couple of million others out there use similar guidance?

We didn't realize at first that this was the seed of an idea for a book because we were simply too hungry for the information itself. It's not that we didn't have dates or girlfriends: After all, this was the pre-AIDS era and we were young and single in a city teeming with single women. But you could say we were sexually unsophisticated. (Except for Todd, who was always arguing otherwise. Of course he also had the girlfriend who did anatomical drawings.) The point was—and is—that as heterosexual men we needed basic information about women and their bodies that for one reason or another had eluded us until that night on East Fourteenth Street in New York City.

Five years later, after I'd finished writing *How a Man Ages*, a health book for and about men, I was talking with Todd in that same apartment. When he asked me what my next book would be about, I told him I wasn't sure. Then he said, "Well, if you write one about women's bodies, I'll help with the research."

We smiled, but neither of us laughed. In fact I thought it might be a fun idea. But I also knew I didn't know enough about women's bodies even to pretend to be an expert about them. And neither did Todd, as much as he might have believed he did. As it turned out, that was precisely the point. What men, besides certain doctors or researchers, truly *are* experts on women and their bodies? Not that many, percentage-wise. And among the few, how many of them want to or are able to write a book on the topic? A women's-body book for men began to look less and less fanciful as the weeks went by.

If I didn't claim to be an expert about women and their bodies, could I still write a credible book about them? I thought so. I'd done it with the book about men's bodies and I wasn't an expert on those. I was a journalist-author who interviewed experts, did research, then explained my findings in print. By 1986 I had written and edited articles about health and sports medicine for *Esquire* and *Sport* magazines, so I was familiar with and comfortable writing for a mostly male audience. It's the subject of women's bodies I'd need help with for the new project. Fortunately I got it.

From late 1989 through late 1991 I interviewed more than seventy doctors, nurses, birth control experts, marital and couples counselors, psychotherapists, psychiatrists, research scientists, and midwives. I also interviewed more than one hundred women and twenty-five men who don't consider themselves experts on women's bodies. And in many cases these interview subjects—the "nonexperts"—were more helpful to me in choosing what topics to include among these pages.

Even if they didn't have all the facts, they had strong opinions about what they believe women want in relationships and in bed. What they want is what you'll find in the chapters that follow. While it may have taken me parts of ten years to get here, my intent is simple: to help explain to men what we ought to know or what women wish we knew about their bodies and minds. And although women may also learn a lot from the book, I asked questions I thought men would want asked, and the answers herein are provided with men's needs in mind. Now in my mid-thirties, having had several long-term relationships with women but having not yet married, I've got a long way to go before I can be considered an expert on women. But, then, this book isn't about becoming an expert. It's about knowing the right answers in regard to understanding a woman's body. Or at least asking the right questions.

ACKNOWLEDGMENTS

In the first few months of this book's life, there were three people who, perhaps without knowing it, encouraged me greatly and who helped shape the chapters to come. Jay Gale, Ph.D., a psychotherapist and author from Laguna Hills, California, whom I met at a meeting of sex educators in San Diego, took the time to explain to me in detail his views of what men need to know about women and their bodies.

Pamela Dunkin, M.D., a psychiatrist from Denver whose practice includes a majority of women, also contributed a good deal of her time—to coach me through the intricacies of psychology and psychoanalytic theory.

The third prominent influence I had the pleasure to work with was Judy Norsigian, a co-author of the classic, *Our Bodies, Ourselves*, and a director of the Boston Women's Health Book Collective. Although my first visit to the Collective was daunting, by my third visit Norsigian opened her Rolodex to me and helped fill my briefcase with position papers and contacts.

I would also like to thank Dr. Albert George Thomas of Mount Sinai Medical School department of OB/GYN in New York City, Dr. Gail Brockman of Los Angeles, Dr. Craig Strafford of the Holzer Clinic in Gallipolis, Ohio, Margaret Pepe, Ph.D., of Kent State University, Dr. Richard Skolnik of New York City, Dr. Randall E. McNally of Northbrook and Chicago, Illinois, Jennifer Knopf, Ph.D., of Northwestern University's sex and marital therapy program, Marty Klein, Ph.D., a Palo Alto, California, psychotherapist and author, and Herb Goldberg, Ph.D., a Los Angeles psychotherapist and author.

At the Sex Information and Education Council of the United States (SIECUS), I owe thanks to Daniel Donahue and Jim Shortridge, librarians extraordinaire, as well as to Executive Director Debra Haffner, who always seemed to have time for my questions about the murky political/psychosexual scene.

In the world of magazines, a number of editors were particularly helpful in guiding me along, including Lisa Bain at *Glamour*, Jon Rizzi while at *New York Woman*, Robbie Myers at *Seventeen* (and at the office), and Kathy Rich while at *GQ*. At *Self*, Alexandra Penney was generous with her time and suggestions on how to maneuver this project through its final stages. For research help that was both timely and rich, I thank Michele Tomasik and Elena Rover.

Thanks also to the dozens of doctors and other medical professionals who took my calls and received my faxes without knowing when or whether their comments would see print. In other important ways, Nancy Duffy, Ed McNally, Jennifer Mitchell, Helene Rubinstein, and Michael Schrage pitched in with friendship and advice. And special gratitude goes out to the 135 women who so graciously agreed to share intimate parts of their lives in interviews—simply to help educate men about the opposite sex. Without them, this book would have been slim. Without Joelle Delbourgo, Lynn Rosen, and Julie Merberg at Ballantine Books, this book might not have been at all. Ditto for Flip Brophy, the best agent and life-counselor a writer could want.

Finally, I'd like to thank Geoff Hansen for donating a secluded place to write in the Berkshire Hills, when I needed it most. To Todd Neal, I salute you for being so enthusiastic about the idea of a book for men about women so early on. It was so obvious, in fact, that it wasn't. To all of you, I'll take responsibility for exaggerations or misstatements that may appear in these pages if you'll take credit for the pages that shine.

WHAT SHE WANTS

CHAPTER 1

WHAT MEN SHOULD KNOW:
ONE MAN'S LESSONS

I met up with Terri on the streets of Los Angeles, and we decided to head back to her place. But first we stopped off at a convenience store to buy beer. We weren't strangers, but neither were we friends.

Terri D. was a twenty-six-year-old, fair-complected friend of a friend. She was also a lover of a bachelor friend of mine, for I knew they had dated a few times and slept together more than once. We got to talking. A few beers later I found out she was anything but shy.

"The most amazing relationship I ever had," Terri told me, "was with a married man while I was engaged. The danger was an amazing element. After a while I could make him come just by talking to him." A little later she said, "There's no greater feeling in the world than coming."

"This is good," I thought. After all, I'd come to Terri's town to ask her some intimate questions for the book you're now holding, one written for men about women and their bodies. For one and a half years this was my job. Besides Los Angeles I traveled to Akron (Ohio), Boston, Chicago, Cleveland, Denver, Miami, Phoenix, St. Louis, San Diego, San Francisco, Washington, D.C., and around New York, where I live, to ask more than 130 women if they would share parts of their private lives in order to help men learn more about women. Most of them were happy to help.

I told the women up front that I was not a doctor or a therapist. I simply said I was a journalist, with a background in magazines and health, and an author of one previous book on men's health. Because nearly all of my interviewees were referred by health professionals, friends of friends, and former co-workers, I knew I would have a high rate of participation. I also knew my "sample" was not utterly scientific in scope; I could live with that.

At the outset it was clear that in the market for women's books, certain kinds of titles were popular: *Love Codes: How to Decipher Men's Secret Signals About Romance; Secrets About Men Every Woman Should Know; What Men Won't Tell You but Women Need to Know.* Actual titles all, but for women. I wanted facts, not secrets. *About* women. And their faces, breasts, hips, vaginas, shoulders, arms, legs, hormones, and the napes of their necks. And sex: how they felt about sex. What they wanted, what they did, and what they didn't do when making love. Moreover, I wanted to know what they enjoyed or didn't like doing with men they had sex with. I considered these interview subjects experts of sorts—experts on their own bodies and on real-life sex. On the other hand I also talked with obstetricians, gynecologists, psychiatrists, psychologists, sexologists, and couples counselors, to research the more scientific sides of sex and sexual health.

One reason I wanted facts, not "secrets," was because a woman's body—in particular its reproductive and endocrine systems—is at once more complex and more variable than a man's. And as one West Coast psychotherapist told me, men don't talk about sex as often, or as deeply, as women typically do. That, he thought, was a major cause of sexual problems between the sexes. It's not that women are keeping secrets but that men aren't getting hold of the facts.

Early on it occurred to me that there was a lot men could learn directly from women about their bodies, from why women feel differently than men about their physical selves to how they wished their partners would caress them. I felt this kind of knowledge would help both sexes. So I started asking female strangers about their sex lives, past and present. I asked them medical questions, such as whether they suffered from premenstrual syndrome (PMS), and questions about such things as how they thought hormones influenced their moods and behavior. (To have good sex, sexologists say, it helps to have good sexual health.) I made a point of asking this latter question because early in my reporting, one doctor, who specialized in treating women, told me she believed hormones "are the most important but least understood difference between the sexes." Throughout my travels I kept those words in mind.

On more than one occasion I felt I'd drifted into uneasy terrain. The truth is, I sometimes found myself straddling a quivering line between sexual confession and what felt to me like subliminal seduction. Sure, I wanted to know some quite personal details. And I wanted these women to trust me enough—as a professional interviewer—to allow me to record their thoughts and feelings. But how far should our conversations go? I wasn't sure at the beginning; I was more confident at the end. To uphold objectivity, I tried to keep (or insert) some distance in even the most evocative of interviews. As the months passed, I felt myself becoming more open sexually in conversation, if not in my personal life. The point was, and is, the women wanted to talk.

One woman I spoke with told me, without my asking, precisely how she moves her fingers when she masturbates. Another woman told me about the time she consummated a long-running, on-and-off flirtation she had with a millionaire she had known for four years. What bothered her, she said, was that he made her take a shower before he would make love with her. "That was not negotiable," she said. Then he brought out warm body oil and massaged it over her entire body.

As it turned out, she said the requisite shower and hot-oil massage seemed so routine for him—so *planned*—that it actually spoiled the sex for her. She told me further that she was shy about nudity and sex in the first place, and the fact that this man didn't pick up on that made her feel terribly uncomfortable. "This is not 'what she wants,' " I remember thinking. Which led to my first invaluable lesson about men's knowledge of women's bodies:

LESSON #1: THERE IS NO SHAME IN A MAN ADMITTING WHAT HE DOESN'T KNOW ABOUT A WOMAN'S BODY.

Eleanor H., a recently married thirty-three-year-old who lives outside Baltimore, wholeheartedly agrees. "There's nothing men *should* know about a woman's body," she says, "because I know how different I feel from time to time or day to day.

"Even my husband sometimes says, 'How could *I* know that doesn't feel good? Yesterday you said you loved that.' Well," she says, "some days my body is very tender, and he's got to be gentle; other days I am totally insatiable."

Fluctuating feelings between couples, and women's own erratic feelings, turn out to be the cause of a great deal of persistent male-female frustration. The seemingly random variation a woman feels about her body can be justly intimidating to a man, or it may rise up unexpectedly one day and stifle a couple who are trying to become physically closer. Health professionals have long known this, even as they search for individual solutions for their clients.

Sometimes it helps to "try" less and talk more. Sometimes a man has to kick aside his sexual machismo and ask his partner for help. "How do you feel?" can be four very valuable words for starters, women say. They also say quite often they would be more than happy to oblige inquisitive male partners. Many said they wished their husbands or boyfriends would break the ice and ask.

LESSON #2: ALTHOUGH BOTH SEXES SUFFER FROM "SEXUAL ILLITERACY," WOMEN HAVE MORE MEANS TO OVERCOME IT.

With all the talk of the sexual revolution, fear-of-AIDS-inspired safe sex, and even the so-called new monogamy, sex between consenting adults is anything but dead. Among consenting young adults, the frequency of sexual relations may even be increasing.[1]

At the same time, men still don't know all they'd like to know about their partners—medically or sexually. Sexual illiteracy, the sex experts call it. And as Debra Haffner of the Sex Information and Education Council of the United States (SIECUS) points out, we can't expect our government to fill in the blanks. Congress has consistently refrained from funding large-scale studies of modern sexual behavior, despite health and sex educators' recurring pleas for such unbiased scientifically gathered data. Meanwhile, government health officials trying to slow the spread of AIDS and other sexually transmitted diseases are still relying on extensive data gleaned by the late Alfred C. Kinsey in the 1940s and early 1950s.

The reason this matters so much is that if health officials are trying to convince you to alter your sexual behavior, and you came of age sexually in the 1970s or early 1980s, chances are your beliefs about sex are quite different from those of your parents or grandparents.

Then, too, in regard to sex and sexual health, more information is targeted to women than to men (Chapter 2: Why Men Need to Know . . .). There is more variety in women's magazines than men's covering sexual health of both genders; there is a national cable television channel, Lifetime, with a lifestyle- and health-oriented programming base aimed specifically at women. And women typically visit a gynecologist once or twice a year, much more frequently than men see a doctor on average.

"The guy I was going to marry," one woman told me, "used to yell at me for getting yeast infections. As if it were my fault!" If men had better access to information about women's bodies and sexual health, or if they more actively sought it out, at least some of their fears caused by ignorance would wane. Their sexual "literacy" would rise.

LESSON #3: THE MYTH OF THE PERFECT FEMALE BODY HURTS MEN AS WELL AS WOMEN.

How can you better understand the body of a woman you are drawn to today, tomorrow, ten years from now? Taking cues from sexy movies or videos won't help much. Magazines for men won't be much more specific. To get to know a woman's body intimately, you've got to find out exactly how she feels about it. That goes beyond diagrams and mirrored reflections and it goes beyond merely asking her.

You need to get to know her body image (Chapter 3: The Female Form). This area of a woman's psyche has the potential to bring her more torment (or pleasure) than most men ever realize. Part of the reason is sociological. This is because women who subscribe to social and media norms must constantly look "appealing, earthy, sensual, sexual, virginal, innocent, reliable, daring, mysterious, coquettish and thin," writes Susie Orbach in *Fat Is a Feminist Issue*, one of the first and most widely read books on the subject.[2] Countless women seek physical perfection, even though it is impossible to achieve.

In the early 1960s the thin, "Twiggy" look arrived with a whoosh. Legions of women ironed their hair, nearly starved themselves, and bound their breasts with Ace bandages to mimic the lanky London model's look. In the 1970s curly hair and full breasts came into play. In the late 1980s and early 1990s the athletic *and* voluptuous look became the ideal. Perhaps not surprisingly, as many as 300,000 women chose to undergo breast augmentation surgery in the late 1980s, according to the National Women's Health Network. And at least 10 million women are affected by the eating disorders anorexia and bulimia. It may seem to you that women in general obsess about their bodies to a fault, but it's likely that deep-seated frustration is fueling the obsession.

A man can do a lot for a woman by asking her about the part of her body—her mind—that at times is at war with the rest of her. You can help her to see and appreciate her finer points. You can also help by realizing she is not automatically (or obliquely) fishing for a compliment when she asks, "Do I look fat in this?" You may help by complimenting her, truthfully, when you think she might feel down. Or by being honest yet not hurtful. It's not about being a so-called sensitive man; it's not about lying. It's about understanding. Starting small, a man can help boost his woman's body image in a big way.

LESSON #4: WHEN ASKED WHAT MAKES A MAN'S BODY SEXY, WOMEN ARE GENEROUSLY OPEN-MINDED.

Men can take solace in the fact that women show largess when listing what they find particularly sexy about men's bodies. "I like to focus on a man's hands," Candida Royalle, a video director and former actress who starred in pornographic films in the late 1970s, told me. "To see how they use them sensually."

Another woman said (Chapter 4: Women on Men's Bodies) that without a doubt it is a man's eyes—his gaze—that make him sexy. It's okay if he has love handles, she added. Still another said she checks out a man's legs, to see how he *moves*; she likes lean, runners' bodies, not brawny weight-lifter types. To each her own.

Women tended to be less forgiving, however, when asked about what they think *men* think about their own bodies. While men may be preoccupied with the size of their penis, many of their female sex partners think men should pay more attention to their stomachs. In fact some women seem to resent their partners for being so outwardly comfortable with their bodies when they have some excess poundage. Yet this is more an issue of fairness than an automatic turnoff in many women's eyes.

"Men are insecure too," said Lisa S., thirty-four, a divorced attorney from the Midwest, "but a little less so than women . . . Guys only seem uncomfortable when they're naked."

The differences between the sexes and their self-perceptions are often born out of early-life gender roles. Despite the march of feminism, today's adult men grew up with images and role models that taught them their body is a kind of instrument. Think of male athletes, soldiers, and action figures: Victory came through the use of powerful movement and athletic skills.

Meanwhile, up until the 1970s, women were traditionally and overwhelmingly raised with more of a body-as-ornament approach. The reality is, fundamental change in these matters won't occur overnight. It will take decades, experts predict, or even generations. Which leaves men more than enough time to recast their instruments or whittle away the love handles—even if their women don't seem to mind the imperfections all that much.

LESSON #5: SEXUAL FANTASIES, IN REALITY,
DESERVE FURTHER STUDY.

What happens when you take men's and women's sexual fantasies and run them through an IBM-PC–compatible computer? I
discovered the answer to this in February 1990 at a four-day
sex educators' and counselors' conference held in Arlington, Virginia.

On the third day three researchers from Hofstra University, in
Hempstead, New York, presented a scientific paper on eroticism:
"The Relationship Between Sexual Fantasy and Satisfaction: A
Multidimensional Analysis of Gender Differences." In other
words, how men's and women's fantasies differ.

Before presenting the results of their study of 106 undergradu-
ate students, the investigators conceded that their student subjects weren't representative of the U.S. population at large. Still,
the researchers reported some compelling results.

It turned out that when the males in the study fantasized about
sex, they tended to focus on specific, past events from their own
sex lives. Fantasy redux, you might say. When the females in the
study fantasized, though, they usually imagined exciting erotic
events they had yet to experience in their lives. They conjured up
"wish fantasies" of the future.

These findings, though preliminary, lend support to a few ideas
presented in Chapter 5 (The Psychology of Sex: Love and Emotion), including the theory that men may take more of a conquest
approach to sexual pleasure than women. Or that, over time,
women will try to construct (perhaps unconsciously) an idea of
the perfect sexual union.

In both instances sexual fantasy is neither a hindrance nor a
psychological trick employed by a sex partner. It's more of an
adjunct to the intimate here and now, a sexual accessory, which,
experts say, is not a bad thing. "We are not sure, though," the

researchers from Hofstra said, "whether more sexual satisfaction comes from more fantasy, or whether more fantasy aids in sexual satisfaction." The important points are that men and women did, and do, tend to fantasize in *measurably* distinct ways, and that the psychological side of sex powerfully affects physical performance and satisfaction—both hers and yours. Unquestionably sex researchers will try to verify these results, to place their study of fantasy more in the realm of reality.

LESSON #6: WOMEN'S NEEDS FOR INTIMACY IN RELATIONSHIPS ARE STRONGER THAN MOST MEN REALIZE.

Because the early-stage excitement of a relationship doesn't last forever, the question many couples grapple with today is how can they once again inject some of the exuberance, the joy, that used to flood their entire time together?

"If I had to pick one factor that comes up more and more nowadays," says Dr. Jennifer Knopf, director of the sex and marital therapy program at Northwestern University Medical School and coauthor of *Inhibited Sexual Desire*, "it's the *atmosphere* of the relationship, where women are in relationships in which they don't feel comfortable. It's as if they're driving with the brakes on."

There is no easy answer as to how to release those brakes, but there are a few that are worth pursuing. One concerns the therapists themselves. In 1980 there were just 7,500 members of the American Association of Marriage and Family Therapists (AAMFT). In 1990 there were 16,000. The membership more than doubled in a decade, responding to the increased demand for counseling. This doesn't mean that counseling is the only way to fire up a relationship that's dragging, nor does it mean the institutions of marriage and family are dying in the United States. Not at all. What it means is that family and marital therapy is moving more into mainstream medical circles. And that the number of *nonmarried* couples seeking therapy has climbed markedly (including those seeking premarital therapy). These are signs that a lot of people aren't satisfied with halfhearted attempts at intimacy; they want more from their men (and vice versa). Increasingly marriage counselors are giving way to couples counselors, and they do share common goals.

One approach they both use at times is to try to get couples to back off from each other a bit, as you'll see in Chapter 6 (Relationships: On the Cutting Edge of Intimacy). If that sounds unhelpful at first, it turns out it's not. Because many modern couples, whether living together or married, got together later in their lives than their parents did, each with a multiplicity of former lovers. As a result their *expectations* of partnered pleasures are often higher than those of previous generations. In addition, as so many of today's couples marry later than their parents did, they often bring rigidly established patterns of behavior (developed during singlehood) into an arrangement that puts pressure on a marriage from the outset.

And yet by backing off from each other temporarily, couples in conflict can reestablish a meeting place in the middle. By "replaying the tapes" of what they *thought* ecstasy used to be, they can get clearer views of their relationships and sexual behaviors as they stand now. They can also get a lot closer as a couple.

LESSON #7: IT'S NOT HOW OFTEN YOU MAKE LOVE THAT COUNTS. IT'S HOW.

Sure that sounds simple at first. I heard it a lot from women in interviews and read it repeatedly in publications, such as *Medical Aspects of Human Sexuality*.[3] But in truth it's more complicated. To arrive at this lesson, I needed women's honest answers to questions about what they felt was the best sex they've ever had. In Chapter 7 (The Pleasures of Sex: Inside Stories of Arousal and Orgasm) a number of forthright women share highlights (and a few lowlights) of their sexual histories.

Curiously, the women I queried didn't spend a lot of time discussing positions of intercourse. They seemed to want to talk more about the preliminaries—the touching, kissing, and holding. And while they didn't use the words *foreplay, loveplay,* or *afterplay* that I'd heard the "experts" use, there's clearly room for more of that in their lives. Of course, it may have been a flaw in my interviewing technique. Or it may have had something to do with the fact that to these women "fucking is only half the fun." Whichever, a chorus of female voices helped put the Big Question of what women want in perspective:

"In this respect," one said, "I'm *very* old-fashioned. I can't imagine *anything* physical with someone whom I don't love. For me that's why sex is called 'making love.' "

"Being in love is nice but not crucial," countered another. "It is crucial that we have achieved a fairly high level of emotional intimacy. I call this being 'seriously in like' with someone."

"What's sexy is when a man says, 'Jesus Christ, I've got to *have* you,' " Terri D., from Los Angeles, says, "and he 'has' you on the kitchen counter. I want to stay up all night, have fun, and do it again while I eat ice cream."

"Love can make good sex great," says Stacy A., twenty-five and single from Chicago. "It is the difference between a purely physical reaction to stimuli and a spiritual experience."

"I think the biggest mistake men make," a teacher from Phoenix told me, "is that they touch you as hard as they want you to touch them. And it just doesn't work that way."

So these are a few of the most-preferred positions. When you think of them from the female perspective, they do indeed happen to be more about making love than having sex.

LESSON #8: MEN AFFECT WOMEN'S SEXUAL HEALTH MORE
THAN EITHER SEX IS AWARE.

Aside from the fact that women are ten times as likely as men to
pick up a sexually transmitted disease (STD) from a partner,
there's a lot women would like men to know about their sexual
health.

"Guys should be able to tolerate things that are not pleasant
in regard to a woman's body," says Allison B., twenty-six, a single
Philadelphian, in Chapter 8 (Health Issues of Sex and Reproduction). "Like yeast infections. Because if you have one, you want
to be able to tell him and know he has some idea as to what it
means, and why you may not want him 'down there' tonight." A
vaginal yeast infection is but one example. Chlamydia, a common
sexually transmitted bacterium, is another. It infects both men
and women and poses as great a risk to reproductive health as
syphilis or gonorrhea, but most men don't know much about it;
women do.

This can be dangerous because men's symptoms of sexual-
health ailments are often so subtle that they are easily ignored.
As a man you may have a minor infection such as urethritis for
years and not be aware of it, even though you may be transmit-
ting the infection during intercourse. At least most women have
regular gynecological checkups, where a forum for this kind of
discussion (or testing) has been established.

Similarly, in preventing transmission of the AIDS virus, HIV,
among sexually active adults, the responsibility for using condoms or other protective measures should ideally be shared by
both partners. In reality many women automatically assume the
lead in setting ground rules for sex—condoms and all—even
though they'd like to be relieved of some of this responsibility.
"You want them to at least ask you about it," said Elyse, twenty-

six, from Boston. "It's nice to know that the support from a guy is there," said her friend Renée, twenty-five. It's also too important a topic to ignore any longer.

LESSON #9: SHARING BIRTH CONTROL CONCERNS CAN ENRICH A RELATIONSHIP IN UNIMAGINED WAYS.

If men could get pregnant, birth control would look—and feel—a whole lot different. That's what women believe; they think men "get off easy" in this area. In Chapter 9 (Birth Control News and Women's Views) you'll hear a number of women talk frankly about how their sex lives are affected by birth control—for better and worse.

"I resent when men don't ask about it," Brigid H., thirty-one, a dancer from New Orleans, says. "And I am overjoyed when they do. I want children, but not at this point in my life. And I don't know if I could go through an abortion."

Consider: If Brigid resents a man for not participating in the birth control aspect of their sex, how engaged will she be in their lovemaking? By contrast, if she is "overjoyed" when a man asks about it, well, who knows what might happen? In the past these concerns of women were sometimes nagging, sometimes burdensome. But in the era of AIDS, condoms and other forms of birth control have quite literally become matters of life and death.

On a brighter note, along with increasing concerns about sexually transmitted diseases, a certain playfulness about birth control has found its way into the sexual lexicon—as well as the bedroom. Inserting diaphragms, rolling on rubbers—these acts often become integrated into foreplay today, when women or men don't mind asking for help (or when they don't need to). The "time-out"-for-contraception becomes part of the partnered fun.

As experienced adults know all too well, the damn things don't magically move into place. They get in the way; they interrupt frenzied sessions of spontaneous sex. So I was glad to hear from women that a little levity and understanding can help the effectiveness of whatever birth control method you choose.

LESSON #10: PREGNANT WOMEN MAKE GOOD LOVERS.

Most of the fathers I interviewed made jokes at first when I asked them about their sex lives during pregnancy. So did some of the pregnant women and new mothers. "We hadn't had sex for six months before she got pregnant anyway," one thirty-two-year-old new dad reported. "So what's the difference?"

The difference is that some of the couples interviewed did their "homework" and used pregnancy as an impetus to have sex in new ways and try different positions of intercourse: side-by-side, rear entry, or woman-on-top (Chapter 10: Pregnancy and Childbirth for Men). They learned from their obstetricians, childbirth books, or friends that once morning sickness subsides, the middle months of pregnancy can in fact be pretty sexy. With or without intercourse. Even if the pregnant half of the couple doesn't feel at first in the least bit lusty or sexually attractive. Somewhat surprisingly, when the editors of *Vanity Fair* put a nude photograph of sexy, quite pregnant actress Demi Moore on the cover in the summer of 1991, it sold more than one million copies, the most ever sold on the newsstand.

In the same vein, one eager father-to-be told me he confessed to his soul mate he not only found the idea of having sex with her pregnant self exciting, he said it brought him closer to fulfilling a fantasy: making love "to more than one person" at a time. (His wife, however, wasn't amused by this.)

At the same time, pregnant women in the eighth or ninth month aren't going to be thinking a lot about having sex. This isn't a rejection of their mates—it's the reality of impending motherhood. Their bodies are strained to the degree that tying a shoe is a major hassle.

So, with a few precautions (including not placing too much

weight on your partner's stomach if you're in the missionary position), and an ob-gyn's assurance that sex will not present problems at *certain* times, the great myth of "no sex while pregnant" can safely be set aside. Besides, as some obstetricians will tell you, some women actually experience their first orgasm during pregnancy.

LESSON #11: IN THE VERY NEAR FUTURE WOMEN'S BODIES WON'T SEEM SO FOREIGN TO MEN.

In the summer of 1989, while visiting the offices of the Boston Women's Health Book Collective, I met a Boston woman named Paula Leca. It was dusk and the office was quiet. I had come to the Collective to look around the library and to do some research. I thought perhaps Ms. Leca could help guide me. After all, the women of the Boston Women's Health Book Collective were legendary in their field. They had written and published *Our Bodies, Ourselves* in 1973—which in various versions has sold more than 2 million copies to date and has been translated into at least seven other languages. In a sense they pioneered the modern art of telling women what they wanted and needed to know about their bodies in books that had both an attitude (feminist) and a high degree of reliability.

I knew that the women of the Collective also harbored a distrust of the male-dominated medical health-care system in the United States. One of the reasons they got together in the first place, in 1969, was to meet and talk about their bodies and how (male) doctors had treated them. "We had all experienced similar feelings of frustration and anger toward specific doctors who were condescending, paternalistic, judgmental and noninformative," wrote the authors of *Our Bodies, Ourselves.*[4]

Apparently a certain mistrust of men still hovered about the walls of the place. When I began to describe the book I was writing for men about women, Leca said, "Sounds like another

How to Make Love to a Woman." "Not really," I said, pulling from my briefcase a respectable letter of introduction from the editor of this book, a woman. I told her I wanted to do a (mostly) serious book, a helpful book. Leca nodded politely and handed me some brochures. However, on subsequent visits of mine to Boston the women of the Health Book Collective softened considerably toward me. In fact they became quite helpful. I took that to mean they thought educating men about women's bodies was not a bad thing, and I tried not to overstay my welcome.

I also tried to remember a bit about their origins throughout my travels. They first banded together as women *to talk with each other about their bodies*. So, although I would spend a lot of time in libraries and doctors' lounges, I made sure to spend hundreds of hours letting women talk into my tape recorder and notebooks about their bodies and their minds. You'll find excerpts of these interviews throughout Chapter 11 (Final Thoughts: What Women Wish Men Knew).

In many places and in many ways, from women's health resource centers to countless intimate conversations about sex that now take place on a second or third date, there is increasing evidence of why the workings of women won't forever remain a mystery to men. Things are, finally, changing for the better.

On a purely personal level you can help accelerate some of these changes. If you rethink your notions of how women feel about their bodies (and why), you may make inroads into parts of your relationship that you didn't think needed fixing. And maybe they don't. But if you have access to new insights that can help you and your partner feel more connected, isn't it worth exploring them? Don't you wonder what might be in it for both of you?

CHAPTER 2

WHY MEN NEED TO KNOW
WHAT THEY NEED TO KNOW
ABOUT WOMEN AND
THEIR BODIES

She got hot in a deli. In what Hollywood reporters and critics hailed as one of the best sex scenes of the 1980s, Meg Ryan, costarring in *When Harry Met Sally . . .* , stopped talking, stared down her lunchmate across the delicatessen table, then began to act sexually excited before a roomful of onlookers and a corned beef on rye.

Fully clothed and with conviction, Sally (played by Ryan) sighed and moaned ecstatically to show Harry (Billy Crystal) just how much men really don't know about women and their bodies. She opened his eyes and ears to the possibility—the likelihood— that millions of women fake orgasms on cue without their partners having a clue. "It's just that all men are sure it never happens to them," Sally says, "and most women at one time or another have done it. So *you* do the math." He didn't have to.

Sally's erotic depiction of feminine deception not only made a few million men squirm, it also marked her as a truth teller. In getting hot amid the hanging salamis, she actually was getting right down to business. It's time to move on ("Ohhh . . . YESSS!"), Sally seemed to be saying (with clenched fists pounding the table), toward more openness in sex and toward better body talk between couples. In this regard she is hardly alone.

WHAT MEN NEED TO KNOW

"This is the age of antisexual liberation," said Sol Gordon, Ph.D., founding director of Syracuse University's Institute of Family Research and Education in New York. "People are using sex to *avoid* intimacy." In Gordon's view, which he presented at a meeting of sex educators, counselors, and therapists in San Diego in the fall of 1989, we've already left the age of sexual revolution behind. So what's ahead?

Today countless partners are cheating themselves during foreplay and intercourse without knowing it, Gordon and his colleagues believe. You may be in love and enjoy sex, to be sure, but you still may be frustrated in bed because you've made faulty assumptions about each other's sexual feelings.

Let's say, for example, that early in a relationship you assume your partner likes her breasts fondled a certain way when you make love, so you touch her that way. If it doesn't feel good to her, she may bristle internally and yet be afraid to say that it hurts—or that it simply isn't pleasurable. She doesn't say anything because she doesn't want to hurt you. And in this way you form a destructive pattern: you as aggressor, she as injured withholder. This becomes part of your sexual history, part of the sexual behavior you'll build on, marred by ignorance and illusion. It's sex that has become antisexual.

The fact that such furtive behavior among lovers is rampant suggests a problem of sweeping proportions involving single men and women, cohabitants, newlyweds and longtime marrieds, as well as those separated or divorced. And it doesn't stop at faked orgasms. From adolescence through adulthood, the problem invariably involves men's ignorance about the reproductive and sexual workings of women's bodies.

This is sexual illiteracy, and it's pervasive.[1] Especially among men, who don't have as many books, magazines, cable television shows, or doctors aiming information at them as do their female counterparts.

"Men—and boys—never *talk* about sex," says Jay Gale, Ph.D., a psychotherapist in Laguna Hills, California, and author of *A Young Man's Guide to Sex* and other books about sex education. "They'll joke, laugh, brag; but they will never sit down and talk about sex. When they do, it's an exaggerated look at it." Indeed.

"Girls will sit down and talk with each other about how sex feels and what it means," adds Gale, himself a father of a sixteen-year-old girl and a nineteen-year-old boy. "I assume it's because boys don't read that much about it." Sexual dissatisfaction often arises because boys take their sexual naïveté with them from their teenage years into adulthood without looking back.

In the Neolithic era of the sexual revolution, the early 1970s, researcher Shere Hite became the second hunter-gatherer. Following the lead of researcher Alfred Kinsey in the 1940s and 1950s, Hite asked women hundreds of intimate questions, then compiled and published the answers in a series of books. Her surveys were designed to capture women's sexual feelings, frustrations, and fantasies. While Hite's work was criticized by researchers for being unscientific, it was also widely praised and disseminated by the media because it opened doors.

The most successful of these surveys was *The Hite Report: A Nationwide Study of Female Sexuality*, published in 1976. It included views of three thousand women, ages fourteen to seventy-eight, and contained chapters on orgasm, masturbation, intercourse, clitoral stimulation, lesbianism, and sexual slavery, among others. It was not meek: "As much as I like cunnilingus," one Hite subject wrote, "I want it to be over fast. I have a conflict about this because I feel it must be unpleasant for him to get his face wet." As it turns out, this is not a complaint a lot of men today talk about in and around the locker room. It was simply one conflict forthrightly reported.

For all the frustration and anger female respondents expressed in *The Hite Report*, though, there were few explanations for why so many men were failing to please their women. (Perhaps Hite was saving them for her *Hite Report on Male Sexuality*, published in 1981 to lesser acclaim.) In fact it took until page 562 for Hite to note in her first *Report*, "There were a few exceptional men." Shortly thereafter she concluded, "In reality, it is likely that men do like physical intimacy and affectionate contact as much as women do but are afraid to express these feelings."[2]

When I asked various women if they thought men had improved their sexual skills in the fifteen years since Hite first published her work, I uncovered a lot of lingering frustration. Nancy B., twenty-nine, an engaging, married financial analyst who lives and works in New York City, said, "I've only had one boyfriend in all my life who really knew *anything* about a woman's body. And he was the son of an orthopedic surgeon."

Pat H., a twenty-seven-year-old artist from Boston who is engaged to be married, remarked, "Up until I met my fiancé, every guy I've been with has been the initiator when it comes to sex. I wish they all hadn't kept such a shroud of mystery over it. It was so *silent*. I mean, talk to me about the Red Sox . . . or something."

Patsy B., twenty-eight, a single businesswoman in Chicago, complained, "Most men I know probably haven't even heard of

The Hite Report. At least not in my age group." That's not surprising; it's even understandable. They would have been about thirteen years old at the time it was published.

WHEN SEX STUDIES FALL SHORT,
WHEN SEX TALK SUFFERS

In her 1987 best-selling book *Intimate Partners: Patterns in Love and Marriage*, author Maggie Scarf paid tribute to the detailed, ground-breaking studies of sexual functioning made by William Masters and Virginia Johnson in the 1960s. Scarf then set about bridging the physiological with the psychological as it applies to relationships. According to Scarf, what people don't know about normal sexual functioning "can, in some cases, cause them an enormous amount of psychological suffering and pain."[3] The solution to these troubles would involve educating millions of married or partnered adults, and realistically the job isn't getting done. Sexologists of all stripes agree that modern scientific data on sexual practices that could help open new (bedroom) doors are nowhere to be found.

Even the revolutionary studies by the late Alfred Kinsey: *Sexual Behavior in the Human Male* (1948) and *Sexual Behavior in the Human Female* (1953), are by now middle-aged. In fact some of the eighteen thousand people Kinsey interviewed were born as far back as 1900; many others *began* their sex lives around 1925. So the "1950s" data still largely in use is in many ways even older than that. No wonder young people today find it tough to relate to Kinsey's findings. They stem from sexual mores of Prohibition and Depression days.

When a new Kinsey Report was finally published in 1990, it was quite different from its predecessors. It also wasn't nearly as scientific. *The Kinsey Institute New Report on Sex* proclaimed on its cover: "This book is certain to be among the most important sources of sexual information for the 1990's." Now, that may yet turn out to be true, and it is a trusty resource. But the book isn't a classic study of sexual behavior akin to Kinsey's original work: It doesn't tell us what ten thousand Americans did with their bodies sexually in the 1980s. Instead *The New Report* is a compilation of questions people have asked the Kinsey Institute about their sex lives and bodies. (It also includes results of a survey that tells us that as a nation we are pretty ignorant about sex.)

"We have to deal with the fact that 85 percent of Americans say they favor sex education in the schools and yet we do not teach it," says Sol Gordon. "We have courses in *plumbing*; we have a relentless pursuit of fallopian tubes, that's what we have." He adds, "We estimate that only 10 percent of American school-children receive anything close to [true] sex education."[4]

Faye Wattleton, former president of Planned Parenthood, goes farther than Gordon. She considers it "an outrage" that major television networks don't accept ads for condoms or other contraceptives. She is incensed that only seventeen states and the District of Columbia require some sex education in their schools. "We adults don't do a very good job when it comes to understanding the issues dealing with our own sexuality," she says, "never mind our children's."[5]

Where does an eighteen- or twenty-eight-year-old man turn to explore these issues? If he goes to the "*Playboy* Advisor" column, he'll find sex questions folded in with relationship advice and medical gleanings.

[Q.] "What causes a woman's nipples to get erect. . . ?"
[A.] "Nipple erection occurs as a result of involuntary contraction of muscular fibers. It can be the first sign of . . . arousal or simply a change in the air conditioning. . . ."

But even here you may find that the helpful text blocks come up short. "The reason I am who I am," says James S. Petersen, forty-two, the *Playboy* Advisor since 1973, in an interview, "is I am the only person in America who can deal with sex and humor at the same time.

"On the one hand you have Dr. Ruth [Westheimer, the famed sex counselor]," he says, "who treats you like you didn't get out of sixth grade. Or you have to be stern and use Latin when writing about sex. Well, I'm not going to do the church thing."

In the recent past, partly due to the religious or conservative views of a number of powerful politicians, scientific studies that would update Kinsey's have been rare and much less comprehensive. When U.S. health officials decided in 1989 to study sex in America anew (partly because of the AIDS threat), sexologists were hopeful. But before all the health agencies associated with the study could even begin to debate about its final form, the study died.

"It got killed in committee," says Debra Haffner, executive director of the Sexual Information and Education Council of the United States. The new sex study never even made it to the floor of the House of Representatives for a vote. "It was [wrongly] seen as a 'vote for sex,' " Haffner adds. Two more studies of sexual behavior that were scheduled to begin in 1991—at the University of North Carolina and at the National Opinion Research Center at the University of Chicago—also got canceled after they had received initial approvals for funding.

"I think there hasn't been a good study [of sexuality] since AIDS happened," says Haffner. "And a lot of people have changed their behavior since then. I also think problems between couples often occur because people compare themselves to some obscure 'standard' of behavior: (1) How long is the penis *supposed* to be? (2) How many times each week do you have sex? (3) How many times do you reach orgasm per sexual experience?

Then, after reading the [existing] studies, people often feel inadequate or oversexed. What's important, I believe, is to show not only the median, or average, response, but what the *range* of behavior is. Frankly," Haffner adds, "I think men suffer from that far more than women do." Haffner doesn't ridicule mainstream magazines such as *Playboy* or *Redbook* for occasionally publishing their own studies on sexual behavior and for trying to sort out some of the sexual confusion. Not at all. She welcomes the attempts by popular media to gauge our behavior. But she also knows they can't help but be biased to some degree.

MAKING NEW ADVANCES

When we look beyond the confines of sex conventions and aging Kinsey reports, we can see a few encouraging signs of change between the sexes. For one, a fledgling "men's movement" is spurring thousands of men to reconsider their intimate relationships, from long-held beliefs about strong/silent/macho behavior to exploring the limits of their masculinity. And even if it's premature to call it a movement, the banding together of men into far-flung men's groups across the country has proven that pockets of progressive thought can at least make a difference in the lives of the men who make the effort to seek it out.

The beginnings of this minor movement can be traced to the women's movement as well as to Yale professor Daniel J. Levinson's *Seasons of a Man's Life*, published in 1977. The recent gatherings of men into focus groups, men's groups, or wilderness trips with a psychological bent has been furthered along (and sometimes ridiculed) by the mass media. For inspiration, men in search of new sides of themselves turned, in 1990 and 1991, most often to two best-selling books: *Iron John: A Book About Men*, by poet and philosopher Robert Bly, and *Fire in the Belly*, by psychologist Sam Keen. Though their writing styles differ widely, both authors touch on similar themes: that men today suffer from a lack of strong male mentoring and that masculinity need not be as outwardly "tough" or insensitive as so many have long held it to be.

When I attended the First International Conference for Men, held in Austin, Texas, in the fall of 1991, I sat in on one seminar in which three men were openly weeping. They explained they were in mourning for the abuse or the lack of love they got from their fathers. In another seminar a man in his mid-thirties, who is separated from his wife, pleaded with the moderator-therapist to give him guidelines to go about repairing his shaky marriage. Herbert Goldberg, Ph.D., a Los Angeles psychotherapist, was honest in response. He said there is no one set of instructions he could provide; that the problems probably ran deep and would require a lot of time and effort to work through. This group session of thirty-some men in a hotel conference room would simply have to serve as a beginning for these men.

Goldberg and other therapists are heartened by the number of American men today who are making new efforts to talk with their women about the most intimate of physical matters. These guys, though struggling some, are trying to apply themselves to partnering, to coupling, to touching. It's not a question of them unleashing the so-called feminine side of themselves, but one of broadening the reaches of their masculinity. They are practicing giving and receiving pleasure—encouraging signs.

Unfortunately, though, too many men never tried to question or open up their sexual behavior as young adults. Their old patterns are now more difficult to break. Other men say they don't know where to start. Nor do scores of newly single men in their thirties, forties, or fifties, who for whatever reason have had to start over again in their relations with women. Men need to know what they need to know now, because their knowledge of sexual and reproductive physiology continues to lag behind that of their female peers.

◦   ◦   ◦

When I got back from the men's conference, I compared the notes and tapes I'd made in Texas with the responses women had given me in interviews I'd conducted before I left. Some of the women *had* found evidence of change among the men in their lives, even if they would like to see more of it.

Betty B., a thirty-five-year-old married mother of one, who has had relationships with and lived with men in rural Wisconsin and Phoenix, Arizona, said, "They [men] are *trying* harder; they do seem to know where the clitoris is and what to do now. But, by nature, they are rough because it's part of their gender.

"Women are softer," she said, "more nurturing. Men were born and raised with different tactile development: 'CRASH those trucks together!' 'HIT that baseball!' 'POUND that nail!' 'Now grow up and be tender . . . and soft . . . with a woman.' Ha! They've improved in the last fifteen years or so—they're getting much better. And," she added, "so have we. We open up to them more and discuss what we need."

Eleanor H., a thirty-three-year-old married attorney from the Southeast, said of her long-ago singlehood, "What was most frustrating for me was to be with a man who would say, 'Okay, what do you want me to do?' " She knew the man had done some homework—hey, he asked what she wanted, didn't he? But she also knew right away she was about to have what she knew would be "wasted" sex. To her it sounded too rehearsed. (To other women, it may not have.) Eleanor would have preferred for men to take the initiative by exploring and experimenting. The point is to get to know your woman's sexual feelings, not to impress her with your sensitized "new" masculinity.

"This goes two ways," Eleanor said of male evolution in these matters. "If you don't even know the problems out there, you are not going to look for answers." Looking back, she remembers her worst sex as being with men who *thought* they knew the problems. Recently one of her friends, who was getting married and still a virgin, asked her if she had any advice to offer. "Keep talking," Eleanor said. "Keep talking."

No matter how much modern men may try, though, they still find it hard to keep talking. Marty Klein, Ph.D., a marriage counselor and therapist from Palo Alto, California, thinks that our socialized attitudes about sex (or our lack of them) may explain our reticence to emote about these matters.

"Think of it," he says. "Men don't say to each other, 'One day I'm gonna have a wife and we're going to have great sex for the rest of our lives.' Women in the past have trained all their lives for One Big Day—when they are engaged or married. And men? It's, 'Well, we all have to go sometime.' "

Then, too, there are few positive role models of good, lusty, long-term sex in the mass media. In movies, on television, and in romance novels, adultery, singles sex, and infidelity are typically portrayed as thrilling. When was the last time, in fact, you can recall seeing a scene in which monogamous marriage was held up as the ideal sexy relationship? No wonder cynicism abounds. Sure, sex sells, but some kinds of sex sell better than others. And because of that, men suffer.

On the other hand, women suffer, too, through bad sex, says therapist Jay Gale, who also wrote *The Teenage Girl's Guide to Sex*, because some men respond to women's sexuality by thinking, " 'There's a hole there, you stick it in,' and their big concern is whether she is going to reach orgasm or not. As long as they feel the woman is satisfied, they won't take time to explore."

What women hope, ultimately, is that as a man you will learn, explore, and ask, and that you'll *want* to learn, explore, and ask. In many cases they'll settle for two out of three. One thing remains clear: The landscape of male-female relations has been littered with confusion and sexual illiteracy for too long.

CHAPTER 3

THE FEMALE FORM:

BODY IMAGE AND

IMPLICATIONS

"**W**here's the *jockstrap* issue?" a demonstrator yelled into the unusually warm February air.

"Women are not a sport!" shouted another, a member of the New York Anti-Sexist Men's Action Network, sponsors of the rally-in-progress. At high noon, on the corner of Fiftieth Street and Avenue of the Americas, outside the Time & Life Building in New York City's Rockefeller Center, fifteen demonstrators were incensed over thirty-six pages of models dressed in swim-suits, posing provocatively for the twenty-sixth annual *Sports Illustrated* swimsuit issue. And while this mingling of sports, sex and Spandex gets a lot of people hot and bothered every year, protestors in the past had never countered with such an odd, angry arsenal. At the epicenter of the rally stood its star attraction: a six-foot-tall penis, cocked at a 45-degree angle, with a polyboard hand sliding up and down the shaft. It took two protestors to hold up the outsized erection, which was aimed at a large mock-up magazine cover of "Spurts Illustrated."

"*That's* worse than anything in the magazine," said a middle-aged businessman passing by. To the protestors, though, the "sexploitation" of women in a mainstream magazine reaching millions of men was far more destructive.

Why all the fuss? Haven't attractive women been objectified for decades, for centuries? "It's not as bad as *Playboy* or *Penthouse*," supporters of *Sports Illustrated* thought. "It's just *swimsuits*. It's not as if they're nude." Yet a number of social scientists, such as Rita Freedman, Ph.D., a psychologist and author of *Bodylove*, believe, "This is not just about models displaying themselves for men. It affects how the everyday woman feels about herself and her body."[1]

How the everyday woman feels about herself and her body.

That's really what the fuss was about: women and their body images. Leaders in feminist organizations (both women and men) decided it was time to speak up—loudly—about a problem that is bigger than any single issue of a men's magazine, one that shadows women of all sizes and ages. It starts, in media and advertising, with the promulgation of fashion ideals and beauty images that are unrealistic—from selling swimsuits to Gap T-shirts to Yves Saint Laurent gowns. It doesn't let up from there.

"Some men truly believe that all women should have perfect *Playboy* bodies or else something is wrong," says Rachel B., twenty-three, a single working woman from Chicago. "Just as men have different builds, so do women. And I can't think of one woman who is totally comfortable with her weight and shape."

Women's own images of their bodies run the gamut from quite accurate to wildly distorted, and it often affects their behavior, not just their feelings. This isn't the same with men, whose body images aren't askew nearly as often.

According to Valerie Buyse, M.D., a psychiatrist from Fairfax, Virginia, when women try to change their bodies in regard to others' standards, it is one of the most self-destructive things they can do. "Because it is an ultimate rejection of ourselves," she says. And because men don't tend to grow up with the same pressures regarding how their bodies should look, they're often at a loss in dealing with these problems of their female partners.

It's not that women expect their male partners to fix their body images if they happen to be distorted. What women want is for their men to recognize these as legitimate concerns and to understand that these negative thoughts may be rooted deeply in their minds. "Sex is really tied up with a woman's self-concept," says Susan Campbell, Ph.D., a therapist who has worked at the Sexual Behaviors Consulting Unit at Johns Hopkins University in Baltimore. "Luckily, [the self-concept] seems to get better as women get older."

Unfortunately, when they're younger, destructive patterns often set in. One of the first grown-up images of female bodies that millions of girls come to know is the Barbie doll. If you were to translate the shapely dimensions of the doll to adult size, they would measure 36-20-32: an impossible combination of an adult female's (full) chest, a child's waist, and an adolescent's hip girth. This, then, is the body countless eight-year-olds aspire to as the ideal. By the time they reach the eighth grade, more than half the girls in the United States believe they are overweight, and most have already been on a diet. This occurs despite the fact that relatively few of them are actually overweight, according to Ann C. Childress, a psychiatrist at the Medical University of South Carolina, Charleston.[2] In addition, psychologist J. K. Thompson has reported that 95 percent of women overestimate the size of their bodies, with the overestimation averaging nearly twice that of their male counterparts.[3]

"I don't think guys understand how devastating it is when they say something like, 'Your thighs are too fat,' or, 'Your legs are too hairy,' " says Janet M., twenty-five, a marketing manager from Long Island, New York. "It stays with you—sometimes for years. I can still remember something my little brother said about my thighs when I was twelve or thirteen.

"I had a boyfriend once," she adds, "who told me I was 'too skinny,' and another one who loved it when I was emaciated. Their views really shaped my self-image." In retrospect this isn't surprising. When you become intimate with someone of the opposite sex, he or she is likely to be the only person who gives you feedback about yourself *every* day. How could that not influence how you see yourself, how you feel about yourself? The difference is in the reference points women and men have in mind throughout their lives. Society has cut men more slack here.

"You know how they say the brain is the most powerful sex organ? Well, women seem to notice their imperfections automatically, and if you feel pretty, you can put them aside, at least temporarily," says Candace R., twenty-four, a single administrative assistant from Connecticut. "I mean, *you* always see your thighs, and unfortunately guys can change that in you. For better or worse."

"The biggest problem I see with this is that women define themselves through men, and that their need for approval is dangerous," says Sena V., single and twenty-five, from Chicago.

"Yeah," adds Allison B., twenty-six, a friend of Sena's now living in New York City, "but even if a guy is lying about your body and how it looks, you love to hear it."

BODY-IMAGE CHOICES: HOW WOMEN
VIEW THEMSELVES

When psychologists and feminists take modern media to task for presenting exaggerated images of shapely female models as "ideal" women, they often point to the two largest-selling men's skin magazines in the United States, *Playboy* and *Penthouse*, as the prime culprits. Far beyond Barbie dolls, they are considered key links in the psychological chain. Yet Bob Guccione, chairman of the board and editor-in-chief of *Penthouse* magazine (which outsells *Playboy* at newsstands), sees himself not as a villain but as a provider. Through much of his worldwide publishing business he fuels erotic fantasy and stokes the fires of lovemaking and masturbation. In a spring 1991 interview he told me he tries to give his readers exactly what they want—seductive images of nude, voluptuous women who possess specific characteristics.

"We feature women with tight bodies who are young," Guccione says. "Young women have perennial appeal. And they perpetuate an appeal that has to do with their bodies being firm." In the United States today, Guccione says, the 30-million-plus readers of *Penthouse* in general prefer "breasts that are larger rather than smaller, large rear ends, and flat stomachs." This is in contrast, he adds, to the preferences of French men, who favor "small busts and small rear ends." (*Penthouse* publishes ten foreign editions, each with its own cultural biases about women's bodies.)

"To this day I still look in the mirror and sometimes think I'm fat," says Angela N., twenty-eight, a striking-looking model and actress who posed nude as a *Penthouse* Pet of the Month in the mid-1980s. "Yet in the long run I finally know that I have a beautiful body. Because in my business, in the final analysis, it's marketable. The world has been telling me for nine years that I have one of those ultimate bodies. Finally I believe it."

It's a long way from Pet-of-the-Month pressures to the *Ladies' Home Journal*, but leading women's magazines can harm women's body images as well. Consider a recent issue of the *Journal*, one of the oldest and largest women's magazines in the country, with a circulation of more than 5 million. On the cover, television empress Oprah Winfrey was smiling broadly; above Winfrey's face and the magazine's logo a different article was promoted: "Best-Ever Tummy, Thigh, Bottom Trimmers." *Trimmers.* To the left of Oprah's head: "The Most Flattering Summer Fashions in Years." *Most flattering.* On the first page an ad showed actress Linda Evans cooing about her new hair "colourant": "My Ultress blonde does make me feel a shade more confident, more beautiful, more 'me.' " *More confident.*

Turn the page, and a model with huge, glossy lips (a fashion statement in their own right) stares seductively at the reader. "The most unforgettable women in the world wear Revlon." *Most unforgettable.* Inside, the table of contents promises that Oprah "talks frankly about her weight loss, her lovelife and more." (Note which comes first.) *Ladies' Home Journal*, remember, is not even considered a fashion magazine on the order of *Vogue* or *Elle*. Yet these are a few random messages American women receive in a respected women's-service magazine each month.

Some twenty-five hundred years ago, classical Greek scholars and artists had a notion of what the *perfect* female body should look like. The distance, they believed, between the nipples of the breasts, from the lower edge of the breast to the navel, and from the navel to the crotch should be measurements of equal length.[4] But that was then.

From Michelangelo's Madonna to MTV's Madonna, the fashion of curves and the female form has fluctuated widely. Just since 1900 in the United States we've seen the voluptuous Gibson girls and Ziegfeld Follies girls of the turn of the century; the thinner, looser flappers of the 1920s; then curves again and the sweater girls of the 1950s. We've seen the thin, braless, Twiggy-inspired shapes of the late 1960s and 1970s; then curves once more, only this time supplemented by muscular definition. Even the classic work of Dr. William Sheldon, the 1940s "father" of body typing with his ectomorph (thin), mesomorph (muscular), and endomorph (round) classification scheme, has recently been judged incomplete, because his models were men. Women's bodies simply do not change as quickly as society's preferences for certain types. And the many subtle differences often defy accurate description.

"Our society has portrayed the ideal woman as being tall and thin," says Lori E., a twenty-nine-year-old married lawyer who works in New York City. "These two characteristics are not possessed by most American women." Are men bombarded by half-as-many messages in even the fashion-forward *Gentleman's Quarterly?* Hardly.

CONFESSIONS OF A TOP MODEL

"I don't know very many women who aren't in some way obsessed with their body," says Willow Bay, who has made hundreds of thousands of dollars by displaying hers. Bay, a lanky, fine-featured model has "legs," meaning staying power in an incredibly fickle industry. Bay is still around, still working in print ads and in television, in her late twenties, after having gotten her start in her teens. Besides legs, Bay, who modeled high-fashion apparel before her stint as the Estée Lauder *Girl*, also has a beautiful face.

But in 1988 Bay was replaced at Estée Lauder by Paulina Porizkova (of *Sports Illustrated* swimsuit cover fame), who could deliver a New Look. Today Bay calls the look of the early nineties "sexy."

Sometimes it takes an advanced-degree social scientist to make an accurate forecast about subtle changes in physiognomy to come. Other times a high-fashion model like Bay, who has an M.B.A., has a better perspective. "Ten years ago I was like average-to-large, sort of on the bigger end," she says. "Now I'm on the smaller end. Girls [new hot models] who are eighteen and nineteen years old are heading toward six feet easily, and have size-9 or -10 feet. Everything about them is large.

"I think that has helped bring about the emphasis on athleticism in terms of the ideal body type," she says, adding that the most sought-after models are *both* athletic and voluptuous. "What's gone on is the media in general have developed this theory that everything's more 'womanly.' What it really means is that there's a different definition for the perfect body, which is now more voluptuous." Meantime, while the average woman of the United States is a size 14, an average leading model is a size 8. Not a small discrepancy.

BODY WEIGHT, BODY PARTS, AND BODY IMAGES

Among women surveyed for this chapter, a variety of responses confirmed that body-image worries run deep:

"Most women think they're fat," says Cher P., forty-one, a public relations executive from the Midwest. "Not just overweight and undisciplined—fat. Even ten pounds overweight is *fat*."

Irene H., a thirty-three-year-old single working woman from Washington, D.C., thinks her body image is screwed up, but only slightly. She used to be "very overweight," she says, at five feet seven, weighing over 150 pounds. Then she lost twenty-five pounds in the early 1980s, and due to that and the fact that she now wears more body-revealing clothes, she says men notice her on the streets in ways they didn't before. Which she doesn't mind. On the one hand she feels she is still "ten to fifteen" pounds overweight, yet she has no problem wearing a black miniskirt to work that rests six inches above the knees.

"Even women who are not overweight and know it—myself included—find something to be disappointed with," says Teresa R., twenty-five, an editor from Illinois. "You start looking for cellulite so you can find out if you have to get rid of it."

While most women tend to focus on their weight and shape when asked about their impressions of their bodies, some who take a longer view will talk about their faces. "I know I've got great lips," one thirty-two-year-old single woman from St. Louis says. "So I use a lot of lipstick and not much other makeup." Others say they spend more time with their hair and face makeup because it is something they can change here and *now*. In contrast to exercise and long-term body-image work, makeup goes on instantly.

Susan Brownmiller, author of *Femininity*, says, "The wearer of makeup dislikes her face without it, believing she is wan, colorless, uninteresting, flat, an insignificant blob of blemished skin with eyes that are too small, a nose that is too broad, cheekbones that are nonexistent and a mouth that fails of its own accord to whisper of sexual desire."[5]

Brownmiller also believes that women suffer psychologically from being made to think that having hair on their body—except for pubic hair—is unflattering and unfashionable. "Beyond a certain arbitrary cutoff," she says, "body hair [on a woman] is a flagrant violation of feminine beauty and sexual appeal, if not an outright repudiation of gender." At least two points on this subject bear mentioning here: If a man doesn't shave for a few days, his facial hair is often considered "manly"; if an American woman doesn't shave her armpits or legs and heads out to the beach in summer, she is often considered "unwomanly." Somewhere between puberty and adulthood she's been made to reject what her body does naturally—grow hair.

"I don't know if guys realize how self-conscious we can be about it," says Janet M., twenty-five, of New York.

"Most women I know," says Patsy B., twenty-eight, a single working woman from Chicago, "are concerned with one of three things: long legs, big breasts (having them), and big asses (not having one)."

It's no wonder, then, that in the sexual dance of courtship the female partner usually totes the baggage of body-image problems. As Dr. Jennifer Knopf and Dr. Michael Seiler state in their 1990 book, *ISD: Inhibited Sexual Desire:* "Comfort with your body is a prerequisite for satisfying sex." Quite often, and for a variety of image-related reasons, we are now finding out, this prerequisite simply isn't being met.

Then, too, when women feel negatively about their bodies, they can and do imagine others feeling the same way about them. "In fact," says psychiatrist Valerie Buyse, M.D., "people who feel negatively toward their bodies scan the environment, *looking* for negative clues. And if you look hard enough, you'll find them."

Playing off this idea, psychologist Rita Freedman says women have "a right" to feel comfortable in their own skin, as well as a responsibility to judge themselves according to realistic standards. What both men and women need to know about body-image problems is that one's body image is deeply affected by one's self-esteem (or lack thereof) and one's actual attractiveness. If distortions are allowed to take root, that person's attempts at physical intimacy will almost certainly suffer.

In one sense, body-image awareness is said to be growing among women nationwide. That's the good news. Even in instances where faulty body imagery remains, women who used to be blind to it are now at least conscious of their distortions. The bad news is that the notion of a healthy body image has also become clouded frequently by new demands of fitness. The emphasis on exercise has intensified the pressure on many women instead of reducing it. As Joan Jacobs Brumberg writes in *The History of Anorexia Nervosa* (1988), "A narcissism based on health is not different from one based on beauty." Meanwhile "exercise excessives" are being reported in larger numbers nationwide.

In the popular arena of aerobic-workout classes, where women outnumber men by ratios of up to 10 to 1, these exercise excessives aren't always easy to spot. Some are incredibly thin, some aren't; others appear to be of normal weight. Some are simply dancing their way to better—then worse—health and will not stop.

Mostly females of the middle- to upper-income classes, these excessives are not addicts in the traditional sense. (Which is why today's sports-medicine doctors prefer the term *excessives* to *addicts*.) But no matter what you call them, these women are high-stepping their ways to hospital emergency rooms with increasing frequency. Stress fractures, broken bones, torn ligaments, malnutrition. Still they *dance*.

Molly Fox, a leading aerobics instructor and proprietor of the New York City studio that bears her name, understands addictive behaviors and says of some of her students, "I've advised a couple of people to get help. But you can't refuse to let them into class. They're like alcoholics. They'll just go to the next bar."

The International Dance-Exercise Association, based in southern California, now at least includes information on "overexercising" in its precertification manual. But there are no rules yet in place for when it looks as though a student is in trouble from exercising excessively—perhaps on the brink of serious injury. And unlike drug or alcohol abuse, overdosing on aerobics is not only legal but often encouraged—while a seductive, thumping beat goes on.

In other extreme instances low self-esteem related to one's

body can lead to the dangerous eating disorders anorexia nervosa (willful starvation) and bulimia (food binging and vomiting). In the United States at least 10 million people are affected by these disorders; most of those affected are young women.[6]

Despite numerous comprehensive studies of anorexia that have gathered good data, its precise cause is still unknown. Researchers have only been able to say that psychological, environmental, and physiological factors "are associated with" anorexic behavior. Yet it remains a serious disorder that can take years to cure and correct. "My boyfriend still makes fun of my 'former self,'" says Sheila B., a twenty-seven-year-old recovering anorexic, who attended a seminar on body image sponsored by Fairfax Hospitals in Fairfax, Virginia, in 1989. "He can't conceive of me being that thin and going through all that."

Researchers have discovered that after the onset of anorexia a part of the brain, the hypothalamus, begins to malfunction. This affects such things as body temperature and secretion of the endocrine glands. As a result, female anorexics may suffer a drop in blood pressure, reduced production of thyroid hormone, temporary cessation of menstruation (amenorrhea), and a lack of interest in sex.

Curiously some people who conquer their eating disorders may fall prey to what Adel Eldahmy, medical director of the Long Beach (California) Eating Disorders Clinic, calls hypergymnasia. It's another name for exercising excessively. They've been scared off the [bulimic] purging, Eldahmy says, but they don't see the problems associated with exercising until they're dangerously dehydrated. Nor do these women view their behavior as body loathing because they've internalized their own distorted body images. And confirmed them, day by day, over and over again.

Again, it may not be a male partner's "job" to recognize such an eating disorder or distortion. But if you see such a condition or incidence develop, if you make your partner aware she's being

victimized by it, it could be one of the most loving things you
do for her. And for you as a couple as well.

BREASTS AS FASHION VICTIMS

On the morning of December 2, 1988, a few million male readers
of the *Wall Street Journal* were invited to put aside bulls and
bears and read about breasts. FORGET HEMLINES: THE BOSOMY
LOOK IS BIG FASHION NEWS, the front-page story proclaimed.
"Breasts are back in style." As the world of commerce turned this
day, cleavage won the starring role. "The woman is back on top,
you might say," Frances Grill did in fact say. Ms. Grill, president
of Click Model Management in New York, added that one model,
a seventeen-year-old recent addition to the Click agency, was
"the envy of all the girls. She has the most developed breasts in
our agency—about a 36C."[7]

Outside of the "industry," breasts play a major but often misunderstood role in many couples' sex lives. You may know that
the chief physiological function of breasts is reproductive—that
is, to provide milk to newborn babies—but you may not know
much more about the actual anatomy of the breast.

While it may not sound sexy, the size and shape of a woman's
breasts depend mostly on the amount of fatty tissue they possess.
From the inside out, fat is not only important to the breast, it's
predominant. The more fat on deposit there, the larger they will
be. And the major player here is heredity, not merely weight.

Because breasts are mostly composed of fatty tissue beneath
the skin, the sexual sensations a woman feels in her breasts may
be less extensive than many men think. It's the sensitive skin that
covers the breast, the erectile tissue in and about the nipple, and
the sensitivity the partner has for that anatomy that make for the
most pleasurable responses. There are nerves and muscles connected with the breasts, but not very many and not where you
might think. The only muscles in a woman's breasts are directly

beneath the nipple and the areola. These muscles regulate the nerve endings and erectile tissue on and around the nipples, the breasts' most sensitive areas, which respond to touch, to cold, and to sexual arousal.

"I think men are scared to death of nipples," says Evan G., thirty, an architect's representative from Connecticut. She adds, "Everyone is interested instead in talking about the vagina all the time."

According to health agencies that are interested in talking about breasts and related topics, up to 300,000 breast augmentations were performed in the United States in the late 1980s. In and around Hollywood, Cher, Brigitte Nielsen, Jane Fonda, and Mariel Hemingway are among the luminaries who in recent years have chosen to surgically add inches to their chests to boost their careers.[8]

Up the West Coast, Lynette Maria Boggs, Miss Oregon of 1989, didn't win the Miss America Pageant that fall but might have won a Miss Candor competition had there been one at the event: She admitted to having had breast augmentation prior to arriving in Atlantic City. The cost of a breast augmentation, or boob job, is typically $4,000 to $6,000. But since the federal Food and Drug Administration announced, in early 1992, a moratorium on the distribution and insertion of silicone breast implants due to safety concerns, a protracted decline in breast enlargement is expected to last at least a few years. Saline-filled implants will continue to be available to women, but more for reconstructive than simply cosmetic surgeries.

Dr. James French, a plastic surgeon who practices in Fairfax, Virginia, says his typical patient for cosmetic breast augmentation is a married woman in her late twenties or early thirties who has wanted the procedure most of her adult life. Interestingly French also believes that of all cosmetic-surgery patients, those who are the most pleased with the results are women who have had breast *reduction*. "They are happier on average," French says, "than those who have had breast augmentation." Why? French and other plastic surgeons believe that most women who choose to have their breasts reduced have realistic goals in mind when they choose the surgery. The same holds true for some postmastectomy patients who have been properly counseled about the cosmetic limitation of breast reconstruction. "They say, 'I feel whole again,' " says Dr. Richard Skolnik of New York City.

The most helpful thing you can do if your partner is contemplating breast surgery for cosmetic reasons is to be painfully honest with her about her motives. It may be uncomfortable and it may bring up long-repressed feelings you both have hidden, thinking you were "protecting" each other. But such surgery demands to be taken seriously, especially in line with the latest FDA concerns about long-term safety of silicone implants.

The second most helpful thing a man can do if his partner is contemplating cosmetic breast surgery, doctors say, is to accompany her to the consultations with the surgeon. It's not to deal with fear so much as expectations.

Long before breast augmentation became a fashion statement late in the twentieth century, author, screenwriter, and director Nora Ephron used the pages of *Esquire* to examine the flat-chestedness of her adolescence. The year was 1972, the feminist movement was thriving, her confessional was candid:

"Here are some things I did to help:

"Bought a Mark Eden Bust Developer.

"Slept on my back for four years.

"Splashed cold water on them every night because some French actress said in *Life* magazine that that was what *she* did . . ."

Ephron eventually made peace with her body, she allowed. And she concluded, "Now that I have been countlessly reassured that my figure is a good one, now that I am grown up . . . I am nonetheless obsessed by breasts. I cannot help it. I grew up in the terrible Fifties—with rigid stereotypical sex roles. What can I tell you? If I had them, I would have been a completely different person. I honestly believe that."[9]

LEGS AND OTHER EMINENCES

Mary Hart, on the other hand, as cohost of television's popular *Entertainment Tonight*, has become a different person partly because of her legs. She has attained new heights as a newsreader by showing them off; her legs have become a star. While she is not the first celebrity to have her legs insured for vast sums of money (just ask Betty Grable), she *is* the first $2 million-dollar-leg woman to do so in the history of broadcast infotainment.[10] Her legs get fan mail, monthly insurance statements, and fiber-optic lighting treatment to highlight their shape beneath the smoked Plexiglas news desk at which she sits while on the air. "The last thing I ever thought was that any part of my anatomy would ever become representative of a show," she says.

The allure of legs to men is an enduring one, with origins both psychological and sexual. In Victorian times a woman wore floor-length skirts, not for utility but to hide the appendages that supposedly pointed the way to the seat of sex. Eventually legs became "legal," and before you knew it came midiskirts, mini-skirts, and flashy skintight leggings for running or aerobics class. For the record, though, men may want to recall the days of the Middle Ages, when men of the noble classes not only showed off their legs but wore padded stockings to make them shapelier.

A "leg man," say the authors of the text *Human Sexual Behavior*, refers to a man who finds a woman's legs more sexually exciting than other parts of her body. This type of sexual yearning for a body part is often termed partialism.[11] Sexologists say partialisms are less intense than fetishes, the primary difference being that the fetish so preoccupies a sex partner (almost always male) that he does not see the rest of the woman's body. In a fetish the body *part* becomes the desired sexual object.

Since the early 1980s the desire for shapely legs and buttocks free of cellulite has sent hundreds of thousands of women in the United States to doctors asking for liposuction surgery. A relatively new procedure that started in Europe in the mid-1970s, liposuction (or suction-assisted fat removal) has grown faster than any other cosmetic-surgery procedure before it. In 1984, for example, some 70,500 nose jobs and only 55,900 liposuction procedures were performed by board-certified members of the American Society of Plastic and Reconstructive Surgeons (ASPRS). In 1986 ASPRS surgeons did 82,830 nose jobs and 99,330 liposuctions (a 78 percent jump in suction lipectomy in two years!). Those figures, by the way, do not include many thousands of liposuction procedures done by non-ASPRS members, such as dermatologists or other M.D.'s who have taken training courses in suction lipectomy but have not completed a medical residency in plastic surgery.

With a practice just off of New York's Park Avenue, Dr. Richard Skolnik says he has wondered at times about how he undertook twelve years of medical and surgical training to reach the point of standing in an operating room wielding a low-tech wand that sucks the fat out of someone's thighs or belly and deposits it in a jar. Yet recalling the first liposuction procedure he performed back in the early 1980s, Skolnik isn't cynical: "I was amazed how much [body] contouring I was able to do with this small of an incision," he says, pinching his right index finger and thumb nearly together. He adds, as long as patients request the procedure themselves—as opposed to yielding to a partner's or family members' pressure—and realize there are skeletal limits to what liposuction can do, plastic surgeons believe liposuction can continue to bring good results to thousands of women who seek it each year. "I sometimes have to remind them, though," Skolnik says, "that they do have hips, that they simply can't look like a man."

On the other hand, with the rise of plastic surgery, female bodybuilding, and "sculpting" aerobics weight-work classes, women today can choose to look more like men than they could have in decades past. (Or, as many of them put it, they can look like muscular women.) They can develop broader shoulders and biceps; smaller hips, abdomens, and thighs. The question is, Will they want to? If they do, will their male partners be supportive? With all we now know about what's lurking behind women's body-image problems, it is shortsighted and unwise to dismiss their concerns as fashion statements. They're simply too important and too personal.

HOW MEN CAN HELP THEIR PARTNERS

If you find your partner or a good female friend is suffering from body-image problems, you are not powerless to act. Start by acknowledging the problem as both real and significant—vocally. Your partner will then know you are trying to be supportive and not impassive or derisive. You can also recognize that besides the societal pressures women face about their bodies, specific physiological changes also alter their self-perceptions. These include such things as premenstrual syndrome (PMS), pregnancy, and menopause. By acknowledging all this, you let a woman know she is not alone while at odds with her body. So she doesn't need to be as defensive around you.

When women complain to their sexual partners that they "feel fat today," you might think they are merely fishing for self-assurance or a compliment. Sometimes this may be so. But other times they really are reporting what they see: a harsh opinion of themselves as viewed through a tightly focused, unforgiving lens. Then, too, although 78 percent of a survey sample cited in the book *Bodylove* considered themselves overweight, 85 percent (of the 78 percent) of that group believed they were sexually appealing nonetheless.[12]

"When I was in college, I was in bed once with a guy I really liked," says Allison B., twenty-six, a single, slim, body-conscious Philadelphian. "We'd been having sex in the afternoon and were supposed to go to dinner that night around seven o'clock. Well, he was a medical student and really comfortable with his body; I wasn't either of those things. What I remember was hiding under the sheets after we had sex because I was afraid to get up and walk across the room naked. I asked him to bring me my clothes so I could put them on, and he said, 'Why? I've seen you naked before. I've had sex with you! I've had oral sex with you!' It was awful. He ended up taking all the sheets and covers off the bed, one at a time. And he wouldn't bring me my clothes. Finally I cried hysterically and he got all the towels and pillows and brought them back to me. He just didn't *get* that I didn't want him to see my body standing up. We hadn't been going out that long and he had no idea how cruel he was."

These days Allison feels pretty good about her body, both clothed and unclothed. She also has a chest of drawers positioned next to her bed, where a T-shirt or a robe is just a rollover and arm stretch away. Allison's friend Elyse, twenty-six and also single, says, "I appreciate it when a guy offers me something to put on after we've had sex. All he needs to say is, 'Do you want a sweatshirt or something?' I might not want it, but it's nice of him to ask."

Besides being aware of potential body-image concerns about nudity, you can (and should) ask a partner what she might like you to do to help with the problem. Which sounds simpler than it is, because if you don't ask, you may end up offering a kind of help that *you* would like in a similar situation. And experts in psychology and weight loss say chances are slim that what you would want (jokes, say, or specific dietary rules) will jibe with her desires.

It's also possible a woman won't know what she wants to do about her negative feelings about her body. In this instance you can take a cue from clinicians and ask her to make a list of positive statements about her face, hair, body, or an athletic skill or dance move. By doing so you can help lead her in the direction of positive thinking. And you can make your own lists (about your body image and hers) to help the process along. This kind of discussion, whether it's written, spoken, or both, need not take days or weeks. Perhaps only a few hours. However long it takes, the point is to get it started and to share it.

In related fashion, as Freedman suggests in *Bodylove*, a couple can break free from the narrowly focused images of beauty portrayed by mass media by developing nonconforming role models of their own. In this way a woman and her partner can boost their own (internal) attractiveness quotients, with or without the help of a therapist. These new role models might be older, graceful actresses, actors, or opera stars, or even female athletes. To take one example, you might think of distance swimmer Lynn Cox, who stands five feet six and weighs 180 pounds. Cox has successfully swum across Alaska's Glacier Bay, Lake Baikal in Russia, and the Bering Strait, which separates Alaska from the old Soviet Union. Have any *Sports Illustrated* swimsuit models done that?

Finally, a man can help a woman in this area by reminding his partner that her problems may have developed over decades. "Most people simply assume that if they just change that one thing that bothers them [severely]," Dr. Buyse says, "that will take care of their self-esteem problems." It often doesn't. The more men who know that, the better their chances of helping to place the body images of their wives, lovers, or friends into proper perspective.

CHAPTER 4

WOMEN ON

MEN'S BODIES

Jackie Macmullen is a tall, blond, thirty-one-year-old woman who gets paid to watch men's bodies for a living. Macmullen is a sportswriter. For eight years, reporting for the *Boston Globe*, she has crisscrossed the country tracking Boston Red Sox pennant chases, Celtics' NBA title runs, and the Olympic dreams of teenage hopefuls. On a typical week Macmullen spends up to twenty-five hours watching dozens of elite male athletes perform. She often ends up inside locker rooms, where players of all sizes strut about in skimpy towels, jockstraps, or buck naked. If anyone should know a good-looking male body when she sees one, it's Macmullen. And yet, she says she doesn't really *see* the naked bodies in the locker rooms in which she works.

"I'm in there because I have a job to do," she says, "When I am in there, I'm businesslike, I'm professional. And I'm there because I want stories, not because I want cheap peep-show peeks.

"If men could walk into a locker room of naked women," Macmullen adds (though male sportswriters don't yet have that access), "some would leave saying, 'What did Chrissie Evert's boobs look like?' Women friends of mine just go, 'God, that must be so uncomfortable for you.' To be honest, I think men are more interested in women's bodies than we are in theirs."

The fact is, when evaluating the bodies of the opposite sex in locker rooms or in bedrooms, women are different from men. And not just sportswriters. In their judgments about men's physiques, women are more forgiving than men are in regard to the female form. They are also more apt to list as important the subtler points of a potential partner's body, such as his hands, eyes, or the ways he moves.

"The first thing I always notice is arms and hands," says Kate H., thirty, a teacher from Phoenix. "And even though I dated a lot in my early twenties, I don't look at men that way as much as I used to. A guy doesn't have to be all pumped up to get my attention. But he's got to have nice hands, full arms. I like them ample, athletic."

"I notice the eyes, then the hands," says Jessica W., twenty-seven, a fashion designer from New York City. "And the shoes."

"For me it's the teeth," says Roxanne F., twenty-five, from Arlington, Virginia. "And when I get to know him better, I like the small of his back. Plus, a good, athletic butt is nice."

"Hipbones are the best," says Alex L., twenty-five, a retail clerk from Aspen, Colorado. "I like hipbones, to hold on to. But in general I just like athletic bodies. And great arms too."

For a variety of reasons (some of which psychologists have difficulty explaining) men tend to be more preoccupied with specific body parts (for example, breasts) in terms of what's sexually attractive to them. As Richard Ryckman, professor of psychology at the University of Maine, has found while studying gender differences, men's self-esteem depends much less on society's ideals of what is "attractive" than women's self-esteem does.[1] Warren Ferrell, Ph.D., author of *Why Men Are the Way They Are*, agrees and goes a little farther: "Each sex tries to get love and approval from the other by adapting to what each thinks the other wants. Both sexes figure out what gets them approval and start perfecting that. Women, their bodies; men, their success.[2]

And yet while modern women say they enjoy guy-watching as men do girl-watching, the ways in which women indulge in it differ markedly from those of their male counterparts. For her part, Jackie Macmullen is no prude, nor is she unobservant. If pressed, she can tell you who on the Boston Celtics has killer quadriceps and who doesn't. But Macmullen, who was herself a varsity basketball player in college, prefers to pay attention to athletes' subtleties of stride, or guile, in action, rather than the firmness of their rear ends or how well they may be hung.

"I'll tell you something," she says. "How many short, fat, bald men do you know who go around with beautiful women on their arms?" A lot, she implies. "But you don't see very many short, fat, bald women going around with gorgeous men on their arms."

True enough. But at the same time, it's not as if *all* women don't pay attention to a well-developed male physique—or the size of a man's genitals for that matter. Some, in fact, are happy to discuss their preferences in penis size at the slightest provocation. With all that's been written in the popular press about how penis size doesn't matter to women, I found it revealing to hear, firsthand, that size *does* matter to them—at least to some. Perhaps this is a window into their evolving sexual freedom: that they are quite willing to say, on the record, that they very much enjoy the feeling of having their vagina filled completely by an erection during intercourse. They may not choose a man based on his penis size, but if he happens to be well endowed, well, that's okay, too.

WHAT WOMEN SEE, AND WHY

As Virginia psychiatrist Valerie Buyse and others have pointed out (see Chapter 3), women view their bodies differently from men. Among men a dominant theme remains: *the body as instrument*. Among women, even in postfeminist America, *the body as ornament* seemingly prevails. Experts say that despite the gains of feminism in chipping away at the ornamental, it will likely take another generation or two before we see real change. In the meantime, as women open up about what they see when they look at men, we can find anecdotal evidence of how the sexes have begun to move closer together, more toward the middle of the instrumentation-ornamentation continuum.

Priscilla Flood, a top editor of *Vogue* magazine, was once asked by editors of *Esquire* to tell 2 million men what women honestly look for when it comes to men's bodies. To get at The Truth, Flood decided to put aside journal articles and psychological surveys. She opted instead for a potent combination of wine, a group of good female friends, and an absence of husbands, lovers, or boyfriends. Interestingly, of the article's 1,024 lines of printed type, only 65 of those lines dealt directly with the penis, which amounts to barely 6 percent of the entire text. (To Flood's confidantes, this sex organ seemed to be overrated, both as an instrument and as an ornament.)

"Women's minds aren't filled with dreams of extra-large penises," she wrote. "Erections, yes, but not monster organs. A lot of men don't believe this, apparently."[3] Instead Flood found that women are attracted to faces, hands, at least moderately muscled legs, and an athletic, assured stride.

When I talked with women about how they view men's bodies,

I found they tend to support a lot of what Flood had found in the early 1980s: "I just like a man to be bigger than me in bed," says Roxanne F., "because I once went out with a guy who was the same size as I was, and when we were in bed, it felt like we were the same person."

"I want men who are bigger than I am," echoes Jessica W., who is barely five foot three.

"But I don't like men who are *too* good-looking," says Roxanne. "I like a lot of imperfections. I tend to like a guy who's a little rough-looking, longish hair, a little stubble, almost dirty, but not really. It's a *look* I'm talking about—not [literally] cleanliness."

"When I met my husband," says Jane S., twenty-seven, an investment banker in Philadelphia, "I didn't think he was gorgeous; in fact he was little (and a little chunky). But by our third or fourth date I knew I was in love and that he was a really nice guy.

"I've only really had two boyfriends whom I considered 'great-looking' or 'amazing,'" Jane adds. "And it was a kick to watch other women look at them when we would walk around together. The first one, when I was still in high school, he knew people stared at him; he was that gorgeous. But he also felt like he was fresh meat to all these people.

"The second guy, whom I met after my sophomore year of college, was tall, blond, and Robert Redford-ish (except that he was from Kansas). He smelled like summer camp—it was wonderful. And he didn't *know* how good-looking he was, which I liked even more."

A lot of women who shared their thoughts about men's bodies for these pages seemed struck by a kind of physical confidence men seem to possess in contrast to their own lack of the same.

"They're insecure, too," says Karen L., a once-divorced attorney from the Midwest, "but a little less so than women. Men only seem uncomfortable when they're naked! [Yet] my last partner liked to boast of having 'the body of a world-class athlete.' He was relaxed when we were naked. I guess I wasn't because of my own insecurities—which he did little to dispel." She would have liked for him to have used one body part better in bed: the part of his brain that governs emotional sensitivity. Then she might have been more comfortable in bed with this "world-class athlete's" body.

Nancy B., twenty-nine, a financial analyst who works in New York, is a body-as-instrumentalist when she thinks of men's bodies—especially her husband's. She's been married six years to a man she used to watch (admiringly) play hockey in college. "My husband thinks his body is a machine," she says. "To him it's full of action he uses to beat other people in sports. It is efficient. He knows how much he can drink and still be in control of it. For me," she says, "it is so different. I don't think my body is efficient. I think of how it looks."

Rachel B., twenty-three, a single woman from Chicago who works in human resources, says, "I don't know how completely comfortable men are with their bodies, though I don't think they are as uncomfortable as women are. I think men's preoccupation with their bodies revolves around muscle."

In one sense this is understandable. For centuries men have been rewarded in competition (and in battle) after adding layers of muscle to their frames. They've learned to put on a malleable kind of physiological armor. When Sylvester Stallone and Arnold Schwarzenegger earn $12 million for starring roles in Hollywood, while John Malkovich makes closer to $2 million per movie, you can be sure the disparity is not based solely on acting ability. Muscularity in macho proportions is marketed to moviegoers Big Time.

Beth P., thirty-four, a married woman who works in advertising in Chicago, says, "With the emphasis in society on perfect bodies (muscles and flat stomachs) and fitness, men think they should look like Patrick Swayze."

"Most men are vain about their bodies," says Cher P., forty-one, a single woman from the Midwest. "Many complain about being ten pounds overweight. But unlike women, they don't exercise to lose it."

"There are times," says Marissa T., twenty-five and single-with-boyfriend, from Illinois, "when he touches some part of me and I think, 'I wonder if he thinks that's flabby?' He seems relaxed naked. Why? I spend much more time thinking about things in me I want to change. Unfortunately I think it makes me more critical of his body too. I've often wondered if other women feel the same way. I'm constantly trying to watch my diet or work out to keep in shape. Why doesn't he?"

Anne G., twenty-eight, a professional dancer from Washington, D.C., says, "I've had boyfriends whose bodies I thought were incredible, and some who were much less than perfect. But the people I've gone out with for a long time usually have good physiques.

"The guy I'm in love with now," says Anne, "is not tall or classically beautiful. He's five-seven, but you can't take your eyes off of him. He's like an animal: his eyes, the way he moves. He's got a kind of animal rhythm." Perhaps because she is a dancer who works out on a daily basis, Anne tends to view men who are overweight as weak. "And skinny men, with no muscle, I consider neither here nor there."

In regard to men's midsections, women clearly seem able to accept some extra poundage on their partners that men might find more difficult to deal with. I asked one twenty-five-year-old single Washington, D.C.–area woman what she would do if her boyfriend happened to have a major-league stomach. "I'd kiss it," she said without hesitation. "I once went out with a guy who had a serious washboard stomach," she added, "and actually it made me feel insecure. Although . . . it was kind of erotic."

Kate H., who is married, says, "Stomachs are nice. I used to like a tight, 'workout' stomach. Now, at this point in my life, it's so unimportant, the whole body thing.

"I like someone who moves slow and easy," Kate says. "In general I like men who are big. It's a primitive thing. You want a man who can protect you. I don't mean it literally; I mean, I can make a living, I can take care of myself. But I like the sense that when I walk outside, a guy can protect me."

"Men who are overweight aren't comfortable with their bodies," says Cathy P., a forty-four-year-old divorcée who works in public relations. "Neither are men who haven't spent a lot of time around women—they're uncomfortable." The key difference here between overweight men and women, women say, is in the moderately overweight bracket. A man carrying around fifteen extra pounds is not going to be as self-conscious about his weight when naked as a woman with the same relative excess poundage. Which may not be fair, but it's the way things still stand for millions of couples today.

"I don't know why," says Joanne, thirty-two, from the Midwest, "but even ugly, obese men seem to think they're God's gift to women."

Lesley Visser, a television sports reporter with CBS who is married to CBS commentator Dick Stockton, says although she wasn't drawn to sports journalism by the athletes' physiques, "I do have a tremendous appreciation for watching the Lakers on the fast break." In the arena of attraction, however, Visser says, "I'm drawn to the Charles Kuralts, the John Maddens, not the Tom Cruise types." She doesn't mind some softness around the middle, though her husband is more fit than fat.

Jackie Macmullen, a friend of Visser's, says, "I'm not that big on looks either. Neither is my husband. Maybe that's why we're together. Every guy I ever dated—not like there's a zillion of them—they were all *thin*. None of them were 'body' people. Now, I don't know if that's by accident or on purpose, but I never dated anyone who was a big football player."

"I am very intimidated by good-looking men," says Allyne B. a once-divorced actress in her early-thirties who lives in Los Angeles. "I don't go out with big brawny guys who come on to me at auditions. I treat them like they're models." In other words, Allyne doesn't even try to get close to them. She thinks their "perfect" bodies will get in the way of a potentially good relationship. Allyne may be too cynical, but as a working actress she has confidence in her abilities to read people (and read through them). "Even though I'm a feminist," she adds, "I think a man should make you feel beautiful."

Sonja B., twenty-five, a political researcher in Washington, D.C., has a different kind of cynicism regarding the male physique. "There are a lot of guys I work with [in politics]," she says, "who throw back their shoulders and stick their chins up in the air, looking like advance men. They always wear the swank suits and they think they're important. Other times you see these guys who work out all the time. Their obsession makes me wonder what's going on in their heads." In a town where power is often viewed as the ultimate aphrodisiac, these men might feel their power suits and ties might not be enough. They've affected a power walk as well.

Sonja doesn't mean to indict all Washington men. Nor even all the men she's gotten to know there. But she's on to something: at times men's thoughts about their bodies versus their partners' are skewed. Other times they're downright repugnant. As Gloria Emerson, an award-winning Vietnam War correspondent for *The New York Times*, recounts in her more recent nonfiction book, *Some American Men*:

It may be true that a woman does not give up on a man because he grows ugly, loses hair, has larger pores, never thinks to wash his face at night, has the folds of a bulldog where a chin had been, if he will only pay attention, provide a life of responses, provide some proof that she still has some semblance of his attention. But that is not usually the case with a male. Because men feel them-selves in peril if they are not pleased by what they see in the woman, reminded yet again of the capriciousness of the penis, they often make sharp, staccato remarks when they feel themselves in danger. Your head is too big for your body, a husband told his wife, who was actually quite beautiful, as if with some good will on her part she could correct such a defect and, while at it, make her legs longer. . . . He might have been speaking to a horse.[4]

Make no mistake: Emerson recognizes a horse's ass when she hears one. Yet having witnessed some men at their best, in war, and at their worst, in war and at home (fighting smaller but still wicked battles), she wanted to wake men up to the apparent inequity between men and women and their views of each other's bodies. When men feel defensive about their physical selves, they may go on the attack against their partners. It both-ers Emerson that when a woman comes to know a man's physical self, vulnerability and all, she may be rejected for having pierced his holy armor. If men were aware of the predicament they unknowingly place women in, she believes, perhaps they would be more forgiving.

As a certified sex therapist and marriage counselor in New York, Stephani Cook is quite aware of the need to raise aware-ness on issues that relate to the body. Whether in therapy ses-sions or in public forums, Cook has tried to help men learn more about women's actual physical desires (and vice versa). In the fall of 1987, for instance, with marching orders from *GQ* magazine, Cook asked seven uninhibited women assembled in a hotel suite the same thing Sigmund Freud reportedly asked at the turn of the century: "What does a woman want?" The answers Cook got were direct.

> **MARY:** "A nice smile, a nice butt. *Flat* stomach."
> **ZOE:** "Looks."
> **CLAIRE:** "No, it's bearing."
> **ALEXIS:** "An air of confidence."

Being familiar with the therapeutic process, Cook didn't change the subject immediately. She knew there was more to be said, that more forthright material would emerge. So she took her time, using the pauses and silence in the room (as well as champagne) to raise the level of confessional outpouring.

> **COLLEEN:** "I'm wary of beautiful men. They tend to be passive in bed. . . ."
> **ZOE:** "Yeah; totally self-involved."
> **MARY:** "Pretty men don't have an active sexuality. Maybe it's a bad habit picked up from being a sex object."
> **ALEXIS:** "Someone who is tall, who has big shoulders, a well-defined body and an air of confidence and intelligence. Does his nose have to be perfect? Does he have to have high cheekbones? No . . ."
> **MARY:** "A good body's more important. You can do something with your body. There's not much you can do with the face God gave you."
> **ZOE:** "Funny, I think men are much more specific about what it is that *they* want physically."[5]

These women, like those I spoke with, couldn't agree on a few topics: whether hair on a man's body is attractive, for instance, or how important the penis or a tight butt is to satisfying a woman's sexual desires. (Most did agree, however, that guys in good shape who wear tight jeans are worth a second—or third—look.) The intriguing thing about these women is that they seem to have been incredibly eager and willing to talk about matters that men used to have a monopoly over. Or so we might have thought.

In one interview a thirty-one-year-old from northern California professed to loving good, steamy sex as much as the next woman. But she also told me she believes women simply don't have the same fascination with naked men's bodies that men have with women's.

"I was young when *Playgirl* first came out," she says. "And the theory I have is that a strange naked man on a page does not bring the same reaction as that of a woman for men. It just takes more for us to get excited." Perhaps this shouldn't be surprising. Many men can and do get instantly aroused—and erect—at the sight of a nude woman. Women, meanwhile, typically require manual contact or stimulation before they will feel wetness in their loins. They repeat: It's not just how a man's body looks, but what he does with it that counts.

"I think men are as preoccupied with the size of their penis as women are with their breasts," adds Patsy B., twenty-eight, of Chicago.

PENILE OBSESSION?
WHEN SIZE *DOES* MATTER . . .

When it comes to male genitalia, Francine N., twenty-eight, a single lawyer from New York City, thinks "penile regret" may be a better way of describing feelings of inadequacy among men than "obsession." If men are not at ease with their physique, she argues, "they appear effeminate. While some types of men's bodies certainly are glorified—the muscular type, for example—most men *can* fit into what they perceive as women's vague standards of attractiveness. The exception is the penis. Boys are taught that there is a strict ideal and that anything less is something to regret." Case closed? Not exactly.

Some women honestly feel that during intercourse, bigger is often better. Carol M., thirty-one, for example, a single working woman from St. Louis, says, "It actually does feel better with a bigger penis inside me. Big is better than small, but it doesn't mean that the sex overall is better. It's just the actual feeling inside me.

"Even though it feels better," Carol adds, "it doesn't mean you want to be with a guy just because he has a big dick. Besides, a guy being big doesn't mean that person is going to give you an orgasm." As she speaks, Carol seems conscious of the fact that she may be going against a strain of political correctness in this age of feminist or postfeminist thinking. But even if she is in a minority among women on this matter, she doesn't mind. "I'll tell you what," she says. "If someone goes out and gets a dildo, she doesn't get the smallest one."

On the other hand, Roxanne F., twenty-five and single, says she represents herself and her friends on the topic when she says, "It doesn't matter that much—really. The only time size is a big deal is if it's at the extremes: very big or very small."

"What's important about a man is the way he is to me, the way he's aware of where I am in relation to him," says Kate H., of Phoenix. "I like a man who is slow and easy. He puts his hand on you, you know, subtle touches."

By the time a woman becomes intimate with you, by the time she gets to know your overall body, and by the time you become comfortable with each other's nakedness, the size of your penis will probably not be a primary concern in regard to your sexual pleasure. At least that's the way most women say they see it.

FROM BLUE MOVIES TO "FEMINIST" PORN

From both a professional and a personal standpoint, Candida Royalle, producer, director, and president of Femme Productions in New York City, has a lot to say about what men do with their bodies. In the early days of her career she used to act in pornographic movies and write for skin magazines that make *Playboy* seem like *Reader's Digest*. These days, in her early forties, Royalle makes what's been called "clean porn," "feminist pornography," or "erotic videos with a conscience." But unlike the old days, she now writes, directs, and markets them. By choice, she no longer stars in them. Occasionally Royalle speaks to professional groups on the value she feels her new erotica has for couples who want to broaden their sexuality but who find fault with sleazy pornography. She begins these presentations by avowing respect for men's and women's bodies.

At one such presentation in February 1990, at the national conference of the American Association of Sex Educators, Counselors and Therapists near Washington, D.C., Royalle was clearly a hit. The conference room was packed. The lights went down. She kept her introduction brief. And then . . . sexy video clips of her feminist porn popped up onscreen. They showed an adult couple, fully clothed, French kissing, petting, and getting hot for each other in the bedroom of an ordinary house. No silken sheets, no circular beds, no crotchless panties. But as soon as the actor-husband started to (literally) rip the pantyhose off of his wife, the clip cut off. The audience, frustrated, wanted more. The next clip, which Royalle said had varied educational (in the age of AIDS) and sensual uses, featured a woman rolling a blue-tinted condom onto her partner's stiffened penis. She did this slowly, to the background strains of soft jazz, lingering with her fingers as she moved down the shaft. The lights suddenly flicked back on.

"Sorry," said Royalle to the assembled counselors and therapists. "That's just a little tease."

In her newer work, which includes eight films over the past
decade, Royalle the Erotic Educator predictably shot scores of
stark scenes depicting male and female genitalia in action: When
couples have intercourse in her films, they have *at* it. But just as
often, Royalle shifted the focus from men banging away at
women and instead moved it toward multiple shots of cunnilingus, fondling, foreplay, and more cunnilingus. The theme running through her feminist porn is that women can get an
extraordinary amount of pleasure from men and their bodies
outside of intercourse.

"What I really think is the big turn-on for women is beyond the
man's body," Royalle says, "though I know there are certain
body parts that have always held fascination for me. For instance, when I cast actors, I like to focus on men's hands—to see
how they use them sensually.

"In fact my most recent lover is a pianist," says Royalle. "He
has a special appreciation for stroking the entire body. I as a
woman, in turn, have made great effort to pay attention to his
entire body."

Royalle riffs a bit more about bodies, and a related theme
emerges: "We're all in this entire piece of skin," she says. "And
we need to know how to use it." The skin as body part. Why
should that sound like a new idea to so many people? Probably
because it's been so often overlooked during sex.

"In trying to identify what's sexy on men," she adds, "it's the
eyes. Not the eyes themselves; it's what's behind them. It's the
attitude. You don't have to be a stud," Royalle says to men across
America.

Men who worry to excess about their erections simply won't
get much sympathy from Royalle. She would rather show them

myriad unconventional images of the pleasures of sex than reassure them about the worth of one sexual organ. "Sex is cerebral; it is really up in the head," she says. "What people should strive for is to take care of their whole bodies. There's nothing sexier than a man who feels good about himself."

MUSCLES, MEN, AND MUSCULAR MEN

Wendy Magson, twenty-six, who, like Royalle, deals with men's and women's barely clothed bodies on a daily basis, approaches these questions from a different perspective: She's a personal trainer and aerobics instructor. While Royalle affects men's and women's sexual arousal through videos, Magson uses music and sweat to build strength, cardiovascular capacity, and better body images. And while most of her aerobics students are women, her one-on-one training clients are predominantly male. In this capacity she gets paid to help rearrange their muscles and fat.

"A lot of men aren't comfortable with the movement in aerobic dance," Magson says, "or they'll be strung out at work and can't put the attention they need into an aerobics class." Fitness-minded men who don't opt for personal (and expensive) training, then, might take group strength-training classes or those in "body sculpting." (Both stress muscular development.) No matter how men may feel about the fat on their bodies, Magson and other instructors say it seems they all want to add muscle. For one thing, muscle is visible. It can be built in as little as six weeks of training. Meanwhile, for all its benefit, a healthy heart isn't as easy for a man to show off at the neighborhood pool.

"It's usually their upper torso," Magson says, "and they want to build up their arms. They want to take the flab off their center. There's this one guy I work out, Jim, who just turned forty-five. When I met him, he was freaking out. Over Christmas he was looking at old pictures of himself in high school, when he was a football star. 'Now,' he said, 'I look at myself and get disgusted.

I've got the round waist and I'm huffing to get up the stairs.' "
For Jim, comparing an athletic image of himself from a few
decades ago with his authentic middle-aged self was more than
sobering—it was depressing.

The trouble is, like women's often otiose pursuit of larger
breasts and thinner thighs, a muscular, V-shaped, mesomorphic
profile may be unrealistic for many men, even with a personal
trainer's help. And unrealistic body-shaping goals can lead to
emotional ills.[6] "In my practice and in general," says psychiatrist
Valerie Buyse, M.D., "men are less concerned with their bodies
than women. I am, though," she adds, "currently counseling two
men intensively—one who is short, the other who is tall and thin
and has never been athletic—who among other things are not
feeling masculine." Bigger biceps and pectorals won't automatically give men added, padded masculinity. What the newfound
girth may do is bring them a bit closer to the body shape they
think connotes a stronger, sexier image. For some men that's
reason enough to do the work.

EYES ON THE PRIZE

The question lingers: With all the fuss over muscles and male
members, can women truly forget all that?

Jackie Macmullen thinks yes, they can. And do. "Once in a
while something will jump out at you," she says. "Like at a Big
East [basketball] tournament, when Michael Cooper was kneel-
ing down at the foul line, he had his back to me, and he has the
biggest thighs I've ever seen. And it just jumped out at me
because they were *so* big. With some guys, like when you see
[seven-two, 290-pound New York Knick] Patrick Ewing up close,
you can't help but go, 'My God, that guy is so incredibly strong.'
But it is only the exceptions that catch my eye." The everyday
body parts pass by her in a blur.

According to one single, twenty-three-year-old woman from

Chicago, the real love muscles of men are found distinctly above the waist: "Sometimes the most innocent conversations and situations are the biggest turn-ons," she says. "You just look at the man and something wells up in you and you just want to grab him. It's something in his look as he speaks, or the emotion in his voice, and you just melt."

And you just melt. At times the Sly Stallones and Arnold Schwarzeneggers of the world can pump till they drop and still come up short. For women will tell you, simply and assuredly (as they have here), that oftentimes when they're in love with a man, the eyes have it. No matter how many articles of clothing their ideal man may have taken off.

Yet even loving, monogamous women take time to look at men's bodies outside of their love relationship. A lasting trend perhaps? It's at least a flurry. In the winter of 1990 *US* magazine decided to answer *Sports Illustrated*'s annual swimsuit sections by running an article called "Treasured Chests." The teaser on the cover was less subtle: "Hunks in Trunks." The spread itself featured six men—four actors, singer Chris Isaak, and race-car-driver Danny Sullivan—in swimsuits, shorts, and wrestling togs. They bared all or just-about-all of their torsos. In any event the hunks were a hit.

"Our readers love young, cute guys—guys who are all chest," says Helene Rubinstein, managing editor of *US*.

The ongoing challenge, and not just for the people who run *US* magazine, is how to define what makes a man sexy or "sexiest." "A lot of it is attitude," says Rubinstein. "Johnny Depp can look like James Dean, but if he's too 'available,' it won't work. He's got to remain aloof. The classic sexy guys," she continues, "are Warren Beatty and Jack Nicholson. And neither one talks about his sex life much. It's other people who do. Their fans love the mystery. What women like to do is fantasize, just like men. But there has to be a mysterious quality." So it may come to this:

Women may want mystery and fantasy in their "stars," but they prefer approachability and sensuality in the men they actually take as their lovers.

"What does a woman look for in a man?" asked writer Priscilla Flood in her survey of the subject. "She looks for rippling biceps, broad shoulders, strong legs, a flat stomach, clear eyes, a firm chin, straight teeth, long fingers, thick hair, and a beautiful smile, on a muscular, well-proportioned six-foot frame. Or a singularity that makes her forget all that."

More than ten years after first reading that, I finally believe it. For women told me time and again of instances when they've come to desire the bodies of "average-looking," nonbarrel-chested, out-of-shape, or balding men *once* they had fallen in love with them. Men's bodies matter, they said, but not as much as their minds. "*Connect* with me first!" they seem to be saying in varying ways. "And then I will find every sexy nook and cranny of your body—without hardly looking." Which is the kind of body-mind development a guy can hardly get from his health club.

CHAPTER 5

THE PSYCHOLOGY OF SEX:

LOVE AND EMOTION

*The real trouble about women is that they must always go on
trying to adapt themselves to men's theories of women.*

—D. H. LAWRENCE

The biggest Freudian slip quite possibly was made by Sigmund
Freud himself. It concerned his view of the vagina, clitoris, and
female orgasm. Writing in the 1930s, the father of psychoanalysis
had a misguided notion of how normal, healthy women should
have orgasms. In retrospect we now know the father hardly knew
best.

In his study of female sexuality Freud wasn't much interested
in understanding the workings of the clitoris. Once he'd decreed
it analogous to the male penis, he was pretty much through with
it. Women who required clitoral stimulation to have orgasms,
Freud figured, were dysfunctional. He believed a woman should
be able to achieve orgasm simply through penile penetration and

stimulation of her vaginal walls during intercourse. Which is how he also became known as the founding father of the vaginal orgasm.

This may be oversimplifying, but not much. With all that Sigmund Freud pioneered, sex experts today agree his biology fell far short of his psychology. A proper, vaginally induced orgasm, he decreed, could only occur after a woman had mastered major conflicts of the mind and achieved a "properly" feminine identity. If the notion of the sexual psyche was indeed reborn during Freud's time, it was not fully understood. Especially, as we now know, because the clitoris was deemed irrelevant—harmful even—to a woman's healthy sexual pleasure.

WHAT A WOMAN WANTS: THEN AND NOW

In answer to the question "What does a woman want?" Freud believed, perhaps to a fault, that crucial clues lay in her early sexual development. But modern therapists are more open to other influences, including sexual solutions that are not rigidly linked with orgasm. Other physical pleasures, from mutual massage to a "return" to petting among longtime partners, increasingly come into play.

"I think women misperceive what really influences their sex drives," says Dr. Jennifer Knopf, of Northwestern University's sex and marital therapy program. "There is too much focus on technique, on orgasm, and an awful lot of emphasis on the quality of a man's erection. What I think needs to be followed up on is the relationship atmosphere. Many women need to feel close to their partner and 'safe' in a relationship before they can have great sex."

"I'd say that's true," says Grace M., twenty-nine and single, from Minnesota. "There's a part of me that holds back for a long time when I go out with a guy. And I think the 'gap' is about not feeling I'm worthy of being loved deeply. I think guys may feel worthy of fucking, but not of having a deep soul mate."

"I think women like to *linger* with their feelings longer than men do after sex," says Renée H., a twenty-five-year-old graduate student living in New York City.

"Men need to know that women love more emotionally," says Sena V., twenty-five, of Chicago. "We love physically with more passion when we're supported emotionally. *And* they should know that women need oral sex too."

In a way, it could be said we've matured as sexual beings in the twentieth century by both broadening and rethinking (even reducing) the role orgasm has in our lives. The point here is not to belittle the psychoanalyst from Vienna but to place his beliefs about women and sex in a more relevant context.

WHAT KINSEY AND OTHERS FOUND WOMEN WANTED

Half a world away from Vienna, at Indiana University in the early 1950s, Alfred C. Kinsey had a different notion of female sexuality. A biologist and taxonomist by training, he decided to talk directly with females of the human species. He didn't try to analyze what they might unknowingly have repressed. Freud took the "why" road, Kinsey the "what." After Kinsey and associates interviewed 2,700 women in detail about their sexuality, he concluded that there was "no evidence that the vagina is ever the sole source of arousal, or even the primary source of erotic arousal to any female." It is partly due to Kinsey's work, and later Masters and Johnson's, that followers of Freud started to reexamine their beliefs about what a woman really wants. They're still at it.

In 1990 Melvin Konner, M.D., an anthropologist, physician, and author, called Kinsey's work "in many ways some of the best research ever done on female sexuality."[1] For Kinsey's *Sexual Behavior in the Human Female* was nothing if not comprehensive. When the final tallies were taken, Kinsey had found that 36 percent (more than one-third) of the married women interviewed said *they had never had an orgasm while they were single*. (Times have changed.) By contrast, 99 percent of the men Kinsey had studied in the late 1940s said they'd had orgasms regularly before marriage by their late teens—by themselves or with partners.

He also found that the number of nonorgasmic women decreased as the lengths of their marriages increased, down to 15 percent over twenty years of marriage. The longer they stayed married, the greater the likelihood wives would experience orgasm. As for how they got there, 84 percent of the women who said they masturbated reached orgasm by rubbing the labia and clitoris. Overall, Kinsey and collaborators found that 98 percent of the women surveyed said they were sensitive to light touch on the clitoris (key point: they said *light*). In contrast, only 14 percent noted such sensitivity along the vaginal walls.[2] Kinsey not only couldn't support Freud's thesis, he fairly quashed it. It was quashed again later when Masters and Johnson did their detailed physiological work in the 1960s.

Like Freud, Kinsey was both praised and vilified when his data first became public. Such is the nature of publishing research about the most private of acts, especially when breaking new ground. Trying to put Kinsey's "new findings" in perspective in the 1950s, social scientists at first applauded his exhaustive statistics, then critiqued their limitations.

When I asked one of Alfred Kinsey's coresearchers, Clyde E. Martin, Ph.D., in 1983, how he felt men's and women's sexual desires had changed through the years, Martin didn't turn to statistics to answer. "I am amazed," he said, "at how well people get along with their sex lives. If you are going to live comfortably with sex, you have got to deal with the disparity between what a person wants and what he gets. Because you can't will yourself a desire for sex." Martin had no doubt. As one who over four decades had painstakingly tallied thousands of survey responses about sex, he felt the key to sexual compatibility lay in a couple's communication about it, not in their frequency of intercourse or orgasm.

WHAT WOMEN SAY THEY WANT

More often than not, young adults suffer confusion before they discover sexual harmony and happiness. "When I was younger, I didn't know what I wanted in bed," says Pat H., twenty-seven, a single artist from New England. "In college I didn't even know what an orgasm was. I used to think sex was like art. You're not supposed to touch it." Now, she allows, as she has matured, "It doesn't have to be like that."

Thinking back to some of her recent lovers, Pat, a fairly voluble type, says one of the things she wished she could have had more of is noise. "The sounds of silence make it real hard to relax," she says. "I wish men would talk to me more." She pauses. "Granted, you can't force intimacy." It's not shouting or grunting that Pat's after. "It's tenderness," she says. "Even if it's just someone saying, 'I really find you attractive.' Or, 'You're so soft.' Or if he'll say my name. I want to see [and hear] his tender side."

In Pat's case the fact that she says she wants intimacy during sex—in the form of talking, holding, hugging, and noise—may suggest something more. She wants reassurance that her partner desires her as a person, not as an object, and that he's *there*, with her, not in his own little world. Not one of Pat's answers about what she wants from a man in bed turned out to be overtly clinical in nature. For her it truly is about making love, not getting off.

"When there's silence in bed," Pat says, "there's pressure." She wants noise from her man, but she also wants to know that he won't leave her without warning. This might be what allows her to relax, to let her guard down. And finally, to feel joyful when making love.

"Sometimes I'm so controlling," says Grace M. "If I want someone really badly, I act kind of ditzy—like Holly Golightly—and hope he catches on. But I wish guys wouldn't let me get away with that stuff. It's like a game I know I'm playing. . . . But the guy I'd do unspeakable acts with would push me up against a wall, grab me by the shoulders (not too hard), and say, 'Are you gonna be a big girl now, or *what*?' I want guys to pass a test; they have to kind of jump through hoops before I'll sleep with them."

Like Pat, Grace wants to let her guard down eventually. But she won't stop playing her sexual games, she thinks, until she finds her life mate. As her comfort level increases with a partner, so does her degree of sexual abandon. "Why else are we on this earth," she asks, "but to be in love with someone, have great sex, and enjoy it?"

"A lot of men out there are selfish, sexually and in other ways," says Laura M., thirty-eight, an antiques dealer from Connecticut. "I've been really surprised by men whom I thought would be kind and giving in bed. Sometimes I've tried to say, 'Hey, women need pleasure too,' but they haven't listened. Or else they didn't know how to give it. Women want tenderness and affection when they have sex. If I'm with a man and all he wants is sex, I go home the next day feeling lonely. Why is it so hard for men to understand that?"

It's hard for some men to understand that because, like men, not all women are alike. Twenty-five year-old Roxanne F., for instance, couldn't agree with Laura less: "Sometimes you *do* just want to have sex with a guy—like men do, like men think. And it's no crime.

"I mean, I slept with a good friend of mine a couple of months ago and it wasn't bad. It was fine. It's all it was. But as a man,

I think he had trouble dealing with the fact that I wasn't expecting anything more. I wanted him to know that I'm as capable as he is—as tough—when it comes to sex for sex's sake."

Isadora Wing, the infamous heroine cooked up by Erica Jong in *Fear of Flying* in 1973, would be proud to hear this. For it was Isadora Wing who introduced the "zipless fuck" to America a generation ago. In short, her mission was to wake the world up to some of women's most intimate sexual feelings, and even people who've never read Jong's novel have likely heard the phrase. Yet Jong didn't feel she could have just anyone introduce this notion to her readers. She created Wing, a journalist—an explorer—and sent her off to Vienna to attend a psychoanalysts' convention (subtle) in the shadow of Freud. But Isadora was and will always be a fictional character, whereas Roxanne F. is real. Even in the age of AIDS, Roxanne is far from alone in her views.

The same year *Fear of Flying* was published, author Nancy Friday released a ground-breaking nonfiction book, *My Secret Garden*. It contained hundreds of pages of women's anonymous sexual fantasies, which at the time were rarely, if ever, talked about in the popular press. Some twenty-nine printings of *My Secret Garden* later, Friday published a new book, *Women on Top*, in 1991, which went to great lengths to explain a second wave of women's sexual fantasies. This time around, the women who shared their fantasies with Friday had much less guilt and much more specificity of purpose.

"I'm the dominant one and he's the receptive one," one woman confessed, "My pleasure is in knowing what abandonment he has felt . . . seeing him change from cool sophisticated male to a man in the throes of sexual release."[3]

Friday went on to say that unlike women of a generation ago, today's women feel it is perfectly fine to express themselves sexually in ways they couldn't before, including lesbian or bisexual fantasies. "Nowadays young women wish their men in reality had the expert tongues of their fantasy women," she wrote. "Men might learn if women told them exactly what they wanted. But women hate giving instructions to the man, telling him what to do, what it is they want; getting involved in their own seduction makes them too responsible, breaks the mood of being Swept Away."[4]

During one interview for this book I met a woman whose sex life seemed to incorporate both zipless intercourse and a wish to express herself sexually à la one of Friday's contributors. Karla D., a twenty-eight-year-old word processor from Philadelphia, takes sex seriously but not too seriously. "Some of the greatest sex you'll ever have is with good friends," she said. "I can't stand people who take sex too seriously. I mean, I giggle during sex. I'm playing. That's how I look at it. Even when I come. There are five or six seconds at most when you're twitching, trembling, breaking out in a cold sweat, and sometimes a man will say to me, 'I can't *believe* you're laughing.' I guess that's why there are so many men with lousy sex lives.

"When you're making love to somebody who is smiling ear-to-ear, it's not just a smile—it's his whole face! It might be a stage I'm going through . . . but I'm still hungry for that emotional release with the physical."

Karla talked a little while about how she loves to embrace a man tightly, chest-to-chest, while both are naked. She also said it's important for her to have sex in different places of her home or her lover's. She likes the feel of strong bodies, and not just in sex. As a former athlete, she feels lean, strong, and at the same time . . . nice. "Do you think about the fact that you still may be five or ten years from your so-called sexual peak?" I asked. "No," she answered. "But it may worry one of the guys I'm going out with. He's thirty-four." She wonders whether he'll be able to keep up.

Karla also said she wishes men were more adventuresome

with her body. For there are times when she feels like having sex but doesn't feel like teaching a partner in bed. When one man recently said, "Karla, tell me what makes you feel wonderful," she said she was glad that he asked, but in another way she wished he wouldn't have had to. I told her that kind of question, for whatever psychological reasons, is tough for the average man to ask. "Trying to come up with an answer is hard, too," she answers. "I mean, I'm not trying to make it scientific."

Eleanor H., a legal assistant from Baltimore, can likely relate to Karla's thoughts, although she's a little older, thirty-three, and married. Still, she was single through her twenties and met many thoroughly modern gentlemen. One of her current frustrations with men's sexual psyches is the need to perform. "They'll think, 'I'll do this for ten minutes, then that for ten minutes, then roll her over,'" Eleanor says. "Are they reading this in *Esquire*? They do want to satisfy women, but I wonder if it isn't tied [too closely] to their ego. They want their partner to go back to her friends and say, 'John really knew what to do.'

"It's like they say, 'Honey, you lie back and I'm going to give you this *present*; I'm gonna give you the best half hour of your life.' It might as well be the fifties, only nowadays it's not solely about the man's pleasure."

However peeved Eleanor seems to be by the state of modern sexuality, she says that these are peeves of her past. She also mentions that they happened outside of love relationships. Now that she's married to a man she loves deeply, she says she feels connections she couldn't come close to feeling in her dating days—even with longtime sexual partners.

One problem Eleanor is still trying to overcome occurs when she is in the mood for sex, and although she can talk with her husband about anything, she feels she just doesn't know what she wants sexually. If her husband happens to say to her (as he often does), "Tell me what I can do . . . to make you come," she can't always give him an answer. First of all, she might not want to come. Second, she doesn't think he understands that sometimes what felt so luscious last night (or last weekend) might not feel so good today. Such as? "My breasts," she says. "Sometimes I want him to really play with them, other times they're sore and sensitive, especially before my period." In general, she thinks, guys don't understand this. And it's not limited to swollen breasts during the premenstrual period. Varying levels of female hormones affect moods (see Chapter 8) as well as nipples, sexual drives as well as temporarily bloated stomachs.

A more pointed look at the sexual psyches of men and women appeared in a perceptive article in the *Atlantic Monthly* in March 1988. In it Ethel S. Person, Ph.D., a Columbia University professor of psychology, wrote, "Some women, as many observers have remarked, *prefer nonsexual caresses* [emphasis added] and verbal reassurances of love and commitment to sexual ones." There are all sorts of explanations for these preferences taking root, according to Person, from biological differences between the sexes to lingering effects of long-ago, unresolved Oedipal battles between these women and their mothers.

Then, too, some therapists think that sexual inhibition may be a result of some women's search for selfhood by diving into romances too quickly or too often. They're in a relationship before they're really *into* it. It might serve these women better, Person and others believe, to have certain achievements of their own or to assimilate positive notions of a number of good, strong women into their own personalities.[5]

Maybe so. But Denise E., thirty-three, a happily married mother of three from Minneapolis, isn't sure she agrees with all of that theorizing. "Sometimes I just want to *hug* something big," she says. "With*out* having sex just then." And while Denise admits she may have some sexual hang-ups ("Don't we all?" she jokes), she doesn't feel a need to dump on her mother or the perhaps unfulfilled Oedipal relationship roles they may have delved into back in the 1950s. She says, simply and straightforwardly, she knows what she wants when she wants it. And sometimes, she is in the mood to hug, to be nurtured. That's not a neurosis. For Denise it can be better than sex. Which is not always understood by her husband. Or by many other men, for that matter, in their love relationships.

WHY WOMEN DON'T ALWAYS GET WHAT THEY WANT

"Have you ever fucked somebody versus making love with someone else?" asks Sena V., twenty-five. "They're different experiences for women; I don't know about for men."

"The act of intercourse is pretty much defined by them," says Candace, twenty-four.

As Professor Person puts it, "The problem of obtaining nurturance [in loving and sexual relationships] does not appear to loom as large for men. And why should it? Women are socialized and psychologically groomed to give nurturance, men to receive it. The [male's] problems have more to do with establishing his masculinity . . . and with the question of whether or not he is powerful enough to fulfill—fill up—a woman."[6]

Jessica Benjamin, a psychoanalyst in New York City, says sexuality has indeed evolved for both sexes, but not as completely as we have been led to believe. The "sexy" woman, she believes, "is sexy, but as object, not as subject. She expresses not so much *her* desire as her pleasure in being desired. . . . Her power does not reside in her own passion, but in her acute desirability."[7]

So women and men do look for different things before they feel fulfilled. And The Question remains: Can you become fulfilled and at the same time be thought of by your woman as a *fulfilling* sexual partner? Certainly you can, but it's often trickier than it might seem.

One stumbling block appears when men resort to "power" remedies when they feel anxiety or challenges to their masculinity. Remember Isadora Wing's zipless frolick? "There is no power game," she said. By comparison, when Professor Person uses the word *power*, she means attempts by men to control the women in their lives. Where does this start? Possibly back in a man's Freudian "Oedipal" stage, when as a young boy he subconsciously may have felt challenged by his father for the affection of his mother. If this feeling of inadequacy doesn't heal over the years (and it often doesn't), it may show up uninvited in a man's adult relationships with women.

Later, then, the theory goes, by "controlling" his adult female partner, a man may be getting back the control he may not have been aware he lost decades ago. "Out of a need for revenge," says Person, "the man reverses his infantile experience: He demands sexual and amorous fidelity while disavowing it himself." When some husbands cheat on their wives, then, there may be hidden Freudian principles at work. Which, analysts would add, is not an excuse so much as a psychological explanation for gender-based behavior in adulthood. (For infidelity is infidelity, despite the theorizing.)

In adolescence most males spend time in a "militarized zone" of what feels to them like hormones in high gear. Zinging testosterone, acne, half-an-hour hard-ons, embarrassment, all for no apparent reason. The fifteen-year-old's quandary. Therapists would label it hypersexuality. Rap musicians would sing about "bein' too nasty to be nice." And it's different for females; it's not as . . . visible.

The problem is, most adolescent males pass through that period without approaching anything close to harmony. Their perpetual state of sexual arousal often remains perpetual, as in: No available partner, *no* available partner. And masturbation doesn't quite do the trick. In time teenage boys may once again slip back into a state of feeling inferior as sexual beings—without understanding why.

Over the long term, then, some men may never be certain of a woman's sexual desire for them. A potentially damaging pattern—possibly disconnectedness—may have formed, although it may never have been obvious.

"I know men can have sex anytime," says Denise E., "but I want my husband to know I could never have sex 'anytime.' I want him to know how I feel, that I'd like to say, 'I have to *like* you [first]; I have to be your friend. Even though we're married, it's not automatic. Sex is more intimate for me than for him.'"

Maybe Denise's husband is fighting his own Oedipal battles, trying to control his wife, who seems to have a conflicting feeling or two of her own. What's scary to her is that she has unearthed unpredictable feelings about the man she married, has had two children with, and with whom she feels very much in love. And maybe his vulnerability is being masked by his attempts to have sex with her, to use his power. And perhaps this is all very normal. So what's a man to do?

"Kevin always said, 'If I can't be good in bed, at least I can be funny,'" Denise says, laughing. "I told him, 'You're wrong on *both* counts.'"

Teresa R., a single twenty-five-year-old from the Midwest, says that sometimes plain talk works in bed, sometimes not. "Women today are not as afraid to say what does and does not feel good," she says. Then she gets a bit more personal: "But when I tell my boyfriend something *doesn't* feel good—when he puts his finger in a certain place in my vagina—it makes me feel like I'm at the gynecologist." Teresa isn't sure whether there's some subconscious battle over control of her body playing itself out beneath the bedsheets. "I think he either forgets what I've told him and continues to do it," she says, bewildered, "or he just does it anyway."

"I used to believe that good sex happened when my partners were uninhibited and eager to give me and receive pleasure," says Cheryl L., a divorced, thirty-five-year-old attorney from the Midwest. "But now there's a component of emotional intimacy required too. I don't know if that's because I'm older and more mature—or if it's due to the age of AIDS and other STDs [sexually transmitted diseases]."

In a sexually perfect world we wouldn't need to read Erica Jong, Sigmund Freud, Nancy Friday, or the latest research from the psych lab. For most of us, however, such a world is out of reach. So, taking a cue from a page of Jong, you can rethink the sex you favor and do your partner a favor: You can do something as simple as wonder, as Isadora Wing did, whether you are always or often "taking" while your partner is always or often "giving" during sex.

If that happens to be the case, does your sex life seem to need restructuring? If it's not the case, could your partner(s) be misperceiving things a certain way? Of course, it's not the man's job to *fix* sexual problems or to correct misperceptions. Neither is it your partner's. But it can help a great deal to rethink what you want versus what she wants, and whether you're both getting what you want from each other.

"It would help if men knew a woman has more nerve endings on the outside of her body than on the inside," says Elyse A., twenty-six, of Boston. "They can learn it by sensing what the other person is doing while they're touching. You don't always have to explain it."

Says Grace M., "What I really want to know is can't guys be nurtured and nurturing too? Because some days I might be aggressive in bed, other days I might be feeling lousy and I want a guy to say, 'That's okay, honey.' But I hate when they say, 'I don't want to get *serious*. . . .' I mean, if I just want to get off, I'll do it myself. 'Cause it's the best sex going."

CHAPTER 6

RELATIONSHIPS:

ON THE CUTTING EDGE

OF INTIMACY

Judged by the standards of women, who look at each other when they talk together, men's looking away is a barrier to intimacy, a means of avoiding connection.

—DEBORAH TANNEN, PH.D.
You Just Don't Understand: Women and Men in Conversation

On the first day of the First International Men's Conference in the fall of 1991 in Austin, Texas, a bearded speaker with a bounce in his step took the stage and asked 750 men, "Isn't it time we saw an age of love?" It wasn't that simple a question. Marvin Allen, a psychotherapist and cochairman of the conference, continued, "I'm talking about a love that is willing to risk something. A love willing to reach out emotionally—a muscular kind of love, a *masculine* kind of love."

"Ho!" shouted a member of the audience. He was invoking the Native American sound originally used to signal assent in tribal gatherings that has since been coopted by members of the nascent men's movement. "Ho!" said another. "Huh?" I thought. I had come to the event as a journalist, not a participant, and I wasn't yet hip to the lingo. But I was struck by the fact that hundreds of men had paid their way to attend an event in which the keynote speaker was talking about how to get more out of love. Allen was challenging men to reach out, to cut the macho crap and *feel*. He was asking us to work on increasing the level of intimacy in our lives, in our relationships with women, with our friends, with our children. He was also asking us to give more of ourselves in everyday conversation—not to "save it" just for the big moments in our lives.

I realize this was an isolated event and that these were in some ways out-of-the-ordinary men. (Many, in fact, were in recovery from alcohol and drug problems; many others had recently become separated or divorced.) But there was no denying it; men will get together and talk about things other than business and sports under the right circumstances. My thoughts turned to a couple of my women friends back home who had ridiculed my journey and the idea of a "men's conference" altogether.

"I don't think women should knock this," said Rebecca G., twenty-three, of San Antonio, one of the few women in attendance that day, when I told her what my female friends had said. "This kind of thing may help their men ventilate their anger, or whatever it is they're repressing."

Like Rebecca, Harriet Goldhor Lerner, Ph.D., a psychotherapist and author of *The Dance of Intimacy*, believes you can't repress things if you want to be intimate with someone. Lerner defines an intimate relationship as one in which neither partner silences, sacrifices, or betrays himself or herself; it is one in which each partner expresses strength and vulnerability, weakness and competition in balanced fashion.[1] But intimacy is more than romance and sex, and it is more than being related by blood or even married. In order to find intimacy with another person, you need to work through the highs and lows that result in a spiritual connectedness.

It is this connectedness that women say they want from men but so often do not get. In this chapter you'll hear a number of women talking frankly about the breakthroughs in intimacy they've achieved, or tried to achieve, in relationships. Single, married, and divorced, they explain how they think their best relationships got better and how some of their most burdensome ones broke apart. Their stories may not exactly parallel yours or your partners', but along with relationship experts' advice they provide more telling evidence in regard to what women today want from men—and why.

A SINGLE WOMAN LOOKS BACK: MARA J.

Engaged once but never married, Mara J., forty, a designer, lives the life of an unattached, single working woman in New York City. She seems happy, but could be happier.

"My mother and father were loving parents," she says, "who raised one son and four daughters with a fairly strict Catholic upbringing." As a child, Mara says, she saw her parents hug and kiss often, but she also got some rather ominous mixed signals. "There was also a *lot* of Catholic guilt," she says, "a lot of repressed sexuality and conflict in our house.

"I always had a boyfriend," she says. "Men always liked me, but I was sexually naive. I didn't French-kiss till I was a senior in high school, when a Jewish boyfriend convinced me we wouldn't go to hell if we did it. I asked one of my sisters back then if it—French kissing—was a sin. 'Of course it is,' she said.

"I guess I projected more sexuality than I had," adds Mara, a striking, dark-haired woman. "I had a reputation for being a slut in high school, but I had never even done 'It.' I had never even seen a penis. Even into my twenties, I was more into flirting than having sex. I was a pain in the ass to guys back then."

Although she considers herself something of a rebel today, Mara recalls dumping her first serious boyfriend in the early 1970s in favor of "a football stud who looked like Superman. And I was a hippie," she says, "smoking pot. We got engaged when I was twenty-one, but we never did it until I was twenty-two. He was going to Villanova [in Philadelphia] and I was at the School of Visual Arts [in New York City]. The first time was lousy sex; I started to hate him. I was young. I left him when I was twenty-three." They never married.

Soon after, she had what she considered "a wild fling" that changed her view of sex as inherently "lousy." "After I bumped off my engagement," she says, "I had my first *real* sex—with a Jesuit priest-in-training. He was an intellectual, a bon vivant and a . . . *priest*. I didn't totally enjoy sex with him, though; it wasn't that great. But *he* was." Which happens to be the paradox that has since held sway over all her relationships.

Mara tends to separate her partner from the sex they have together—because the thrill of it never lasts—and somehow it makes sense for her that way. She loves "the trimmings" of sex, the chase. But she also has long felt something missing in her sex life, something she is still trying, at forty, to hone in on.

"The bottom line is that fucking for me is never that fulfilling. And I'm not the only woman who feels that way, believe me." She thinks back to the priest: "He was a God-damned poet," she says. One time they went to a cabin in the woods of upstate New York. They were out in the woods, the night was clear, there was smoke from the fireplace nearby. It didn't take them long to think: "Let's make love out on the grassy knoll." And yet, Mara says, "The bottom line is: I [still] don't enjoy intercourse that much. Let's *rub*, I always think to myself.

"With my last boyfriend—and this was a problem—when we went to bed at night, I was not allowed to kiss and hug him unless

I 'agreed' to go farther. He claimed he couldn't hold back, that his dick would take over. He said, 'I *can't* just hug.' I don't buy that. On the other hand I'd be feeling affection-starved, not sex-starved. I guess I just didn't feel at the time that it was my choice." So she would wind up "giving in" to sex in order to get affection.

Mara also knows enough about her past relationships to understand the patterns she gets into, her "lovemaps," as sexologists would call them. "In the first year it is always very sexual, very amorous," she says. "In the second year things start to get weird; there is less of that sexuality, less of that lust. By the third year I know it's time to move on."

FINDING PATTERNS IN RELATIONSHIPS

"I'd like to change the way I act in relationships," she says. "But I am a romantic. The next one, well, he's always what the former one wasn't.

"Tom, the last guy I was with, was fascinating. But I knew his stories. I don't understand why so many women get into this whole idea of being with someone and settling *down*. I don't understand why I should think marriage would change my life and make it perfect. I go out with people sometimes I know I can't get seriously involved with. I know I go into dead-end situations. But the first year is so ro*man*tic!"

When reading case histories such as Mara's and those that follow, one thought to keep in mind is that while people have tendencies to repeat familiar and/or familial behavior, they are not doomed to repeat it. A tendency is a predisposition, not an inexorable outcome. And recognition of these behaviors is a significant first step in doing something about them.

Christopher Dare, founder of the Tavistock Institute for Marital Studies, and social worker Lilu Pincus have found that patterns such as these "are motivated by . . . unconscious fantasy and derived from the way earlier needs were satisfied." In other words these tendencies are not all one's own doing. Sometimes in relationships the repetitive aspect of partnership is stunningly literal, as when a woman whose childhood was fractured by her father's alcoholism marries an alcoholic, then divorces him and gets herself into a similar situation once more.[2]

"As a woman in New York City," Mara says, looking back one more time, "if I'd meet a man in a club, we would maybe grind while we were there, but I wouldn't sleep with him on a first date. I usually was there because I just wanted to put on a sex-bomb outfit and dance. Nothing more. In relationships I'm into staying home and purring. But with all the men I've been seriously involved with, their underwear wasn't all at my place. I guess I always wanted some space."

Mara keeps her home decidedly hers and in doing so, she remains part of the huge demographic trend the U.S. government hasn't yet found a way to measure: the *almost*-living-together. In the end, you see, Mara doesn't want her men moving all the way into her home. Or, for that matter, her life. She wants love, she loves great sex, but she wants her own space more. What men need to know here is that Mara's thinking—her way of living with men—is not a New York phenomenon. Across the United States Mara is anything but alone. Women today not only want autonomy and intimacy within the same relationship, they are demanding it. And until they find it, unlike women of past generations, millions of them will remain single.

While every couple supposedly strives for it, intimacy can be detrimental, dangerous even, to those who aren't prepared to deal with its wide-ranging effects. Moreover, attempts by one partner to force intimacy may even sabotage a relationship that is not sufficiently grounded to handle its demands.

In the end, intimacy can be a responsibility as well as a goal. For Mara it remains a hidden goal, one that hasn't yet been realized. But while it is both powerful and a positive force for many, intimacy is not for everybody. Even top-rung therapists sometimes forget that.

THE LIVING TOGETHER–"EMPTY NEST" SYNDROME: AMY K.

Amy K. is single, thirty-two, pretty, and pretty honest. She likes her life all right, working in a restaurant not far from where she grew up in New England, but her love life? She's not as happy about that. She willingly takes part of the blame for the failure of her most recent relationships, but she knows there's more to the story. It's not all about intimacy either.

"I knew when I was twelve years old that my mother was in a lousy marriage," Amy says. "She fought a lot with my father, and he was never around. When he was around, he didn't act like he was part of the family. I remember crying myself to sleep one time when my parents were fighting really badly, thinking of my mother, 'This woman is crazy for staying with him. We could find somewhere else to live, she could find someone else.'

"When I finally asked her (when I was older) why she stayed with him, she said, 'I didn't want to break up the family. Now I'm just too old to leave him. I'm fifty-nine.' Now that the kids are all gone," Amy says, "my parents are actually comfortable together. They fit like an old shoe. She sleeps in the other room, and my dad goes away a lot on his own, hunting and fishing. But I still think, 'What's the point of your life?'

"I thought about that when my high school boyfriend asked me to marry him when he was nineteen—just back from the army. He had cheated on me when we were in high school; I knew he'd even slept with my *sister*. That's when I first thought I didn't want to marry someone who might treat me badly, like my mother did. My sister, though, ended up going out with two guys who hit her. When you come from a dysfunctional family," Amy says, "I think you tend to go after men who are screwed up. It may not be conscious, but you seek out that same feeling you had as a child."

HOW A DYSFUNCTIONAL FAMILY AFFECTS RELATIONSHIPS

The fact that Amy believes this, and is aware of it, may be one reason she so far has chosen to stay single. She says her last few serious relationships have been with men she knew from the start she wouldn't marry. Nonetheless she stayed with them. "My mom married my father even though she was in love with someone else," she says.

Harriet Lerner, Ph.D., and psychologists in general, say mothers often let their daughters down because they themselves have lived with impossible expectations about their roles as mothers.[3] Especially mothers who have raised children from the 1960s through the 1980s, when sexual mores were turned upside down and sideways. Marvin Allen said similar things about fathers and sons at the International Men's Conference in Austin.

"When I met and went out with my first serious boyfriend," Amy says, "I knew we weren't going to get married. But Tim and I were together five years and lived together for two. And I knew he would cheat on me and I let him.

"The guy I left Tim for, Mark, I went out with for six years. I knew right away we would never get married either. But it didn't matter. After we broke up, I realized I was always 'Tim's girlfriend,' or 'Mark's girlfriend,' but I was never Amy.

"I always tried to create the perfect home, but a perfect home can't exist without a good solid relationship at the beginning," she acknowledges. "I was doing it all backward. I thought by making the *place* clean and tidy we would somehow get closer.

I guess I didn't think I was important at the time, that I would take care of myself and my needs after the relationship got going the way I wanted it to."

ON PUTTING HERSELF FIRST

Since her last serious relationship ended, Amy has begun to think more of herself and her own needs. She's seen three of her sisters get married, with mixed results, and she knows a lot of their discomfort has come from their subservience to their mates. So maybe, she thinks, she's even tougher on men today than she really needs to be. "I was hurt badly in my last relationship," she tells me, "and I'm at a point in my life where I think, 'If I'm alone, fine.' "

"When I was with Mark," she says, "we never discussed getting married. Our future. From my end there was a threat there—of 'the monster' coming. As long as you live from day to day, I thought, it's *safe*. I must have known there was trouble underneath. . . . But as long as we didn't confront those monsters, I thought things would be okay."

For Amy, as with many women who have separated from married or longtime live-in partners, gaining a stronger sense of self is crucial to her psychological and emotional development. And as she acknowledges, if this seems harsh or selfish, or if she seems "bitchy" to some people, that will have to do. She says she knows now what she needs to do for herself, and if she doesn't allow herself that, she won't be able to forge an intimate relationship with anyone else.

Harriet Lerner, among others, would agree. "Paradoxically," she writes, "we cannot navigate clearly within a relationship unless we can live without it."

Amy adds, "I've always been with men whose lives revolve around themselves. After two or three months they became the important central figure in our relationship. I didn't think they took enough of an interest in *my* life, in what I want to do. Now I'm looking for someone who's very equal. And if I'm going to live with someone again, we'd better be headed in the direction of marriage."

Interestingly, Amy says she thinks she is more intimate with her friends than with her lovers. She also thinks that may be what's wrong with a lot of relationships today: a distinct fear of intimacy on one partner's part (*not* always the man's). She knows she's been guilty of this, quite recently in fact. But she hopes this is a temporary affliction, a result of her last painful breakup. She wants to move on, she says, both passionately and openly. It's just that she won't allow herself to be swept along in a direction she hasn't had a hand in choosing. No, she has had quite enough of that already.

As a single female in her early thirties who has never married, Amy typifies a large number of women who, in their twenties, lived with a couple of men and who already have had vastly different love lives than their mothers. To many of these women sex isn't nearly so mysterious or scary (fears of AIDS notwithstanding) as it seemed to past generations.

It will be intriguing, to say the least, to see how these women— who find themselves at the crossroads of liberation, love, feminism, and femininity—fare in relationships over the *next* twenty years. For these are women who want, en route to "having it all," to make sure that they have fun, too. In the meantime their partners may be in for a rude awakening. Or perhaps a pleasant surprise—if they're fortunate enough to know what's coming.

LIFTING ROADBLOCKS TO INTIMACY

Self-worth inside and outside a relationship has been a problem for both Mara and Amy, and it obviously has affected how close they can truly feel to the men in their lives. In their cases they readily admit to pushing men away at certain times, even though they say they very much want to connect with a man . . . eventually. I heard similar themes repeated at the International Men's Conference throughout the three-day weekend, and the men who were searching for answers at times seemed angry as hell. They felt they had been taken, both spiritually and psychologically, by ex-wives or ex-girlfriends, and they wanted to protect themselves in the future.

But the answers aren't always neat and clean. "My wife says I'm cold and unfeeling and that my kids hate me," one man confessed in a small-group seminar. "I've been working hard, weekends, nights, whatever, to support them, and I thought I was being a good husband and father. What can I do to change things?" Herb Goldberg, Ph.D., a psychotherapist and seminar leader, was honest, if not overly optimistic, in response. He said what went wrong here was likely the result of years of conditioning and unrealistic expectations on both sides and that it would take a long time to go from disconnected to "whole" and intimate.

Goldberg added that it would take work and a redefining of the relationship. As an observer in the room, I was heartened by Goldberg's honesty. I later picked up a book he had written back in 1983, *The New Male-Female Relationship*, and found a passage that might have assuaged the frustrations of Goldberg's questioner:

> What she really wants is not intimacy but the fulfillment of her need to define her identity through him, to be taken care of and protected, and to have her sexuality legitimized by a "committed" relationship. . . . As a result . . . the male is left with guilt, self-doubt and self-hatred as he accuses himself and is accused by others of an inability to be loving.[4]

Sometimes women do want intimacy, sometimes they only think they want it. The same goes for men, although we don't express the former need as often or as publicly. What Mara, Amy, and others can teach us about getting closer is that years of upbringing, dating, and adult relationships cannot be undone in the course of a few interviews or a weekend seminar. But that is enough time to think about the need for intimate relationships in your life and to realize that intimacy starts not with someone else but with yourself.

A MARRIED WOMAN'S GREAT EXPECTATIONS: ELEANOR H.

With a Southern upbringing, Ivy League education, and lofty career goals, Eleanor H., thirty-three, spent most of her twenties as a single, professional woman in a hurry. Except, that is, when it came to marriage. Recently married, however, she's begun to settle in, if not quite settle down. She now works as a business consultant, while her husband works with computers.

In her personal life Eleanor has had live-in relationships, one-night stands, and has lived alone for a time in Charleston, South Carolina. And yet, before meeting her husband, she felt incredibly frustrated by the lack of intimate communication between her partners and herself. She's a modern woman who knows what she wants and is, at last, wedded to him.

Describing the kind of man she was drawn to for a long while before she married, Eleanor says, "He had to be sensitive . . . attuned." She pauses to consider her use of the word *sensitive*. She knows the language of relationships can be loaded. So when she says she wants a man who's "sensitive" and "attuned," it means much more to her than a partner who merely pays her attention.

"It involves getting out of yourself," she says, echoing what various therapists say modern men have a tough time doing.

"And it means knowing what the other person in the relationship wants at a particular time." It could be emotional support, sex, sympathy about work-related or family pressures, or on occasion simply a compliment. For Eleanor, it took twelve years of adult dating and relationships to realize that it's not only all right to want and demand these things from a man, it's necessary for a lifelong relationship to take root. The trouble, she says, was that she was so concerned for so long about being supportive in relationships that she settled for men who joined her in partnership and in bed—but not in mind. Now she can finally relax. She's in love with her husband. And so far the sex is great.

"One of my biggest gripes about men I've been with," Eleanor says, "is with guys who do want to 'satisfy' the woman, but it's like, 'Honey, you just lie back and I'm going to give you this present.' I must admit, though," she adds, "these experiences all happened to me outside of love relationships. A man has to know, even though this sounds obvious, that he should *listen* to his woman. And not just in bed." Esteemed marital therapists have said for years that men in general could do a better job of listening, but when Eleanor says this, it rings true with experience. She has dated and lived with a variety of men; she's "listened" a lot, too. And she admits she's made mistakes.

"With this one guy I knew," Eleanor says, "we were friends for a long time, until he wanted to make it sexual. And there's nothing wrong with sexual tension. Before he brought it up, I was thinking, 'If he wants to go to bed with me, I'd say all right.' But I also thought if *I* pushed it, it could end up being uncomfortable. Then I'd blame myself."

It turns out Eleanor did have sex with this longtime friend and she later had second thoughts. Not about the sex per se, but about the fact that they couldn't talk about the stirring sexual feelings they had for each other. It was one thing to be friends feeling sexual tension and quite another to be friends who had become sexual partners. Is there such a thing as a halfhearted orgasm? "I was responding too quickly," Eleanor says, not quite answering the question, "but I hated the awkward feelings that followed. 'Hey, we're grown-ups. Let's decide this. Are we going to bed or not?' "

Eleanor learned, though. She now says that maybe she needed mistakes like this to help her realize when a potential life partner had indeed entered her life. Years later, when she met the man who became her husband, she held back at first when similar thoughts of sex floated in the unsettled air about them. "I knew enough about myself at this point," she says. "So I was going to sit on my hands this time." They took their time getting into the sexual part of their relationship, even though this was the late 1980s and they'd both lived through the free-love decade before as single adults. Or perhaps *because* of that, they didn't want to rush into what they'd both found frustrating so often before.

In time, nurtured but not driven by sex, their relationship flourished. Looking back, Eleanor realizes that waiting two months to have intercourse with a boyfriend wouldn't have seemed strange to women of previous generations. And she's not saying all men should wait, wait, wait before making love with potential mates. She simply believes the wait worked well for both of them in this instance because they had a chance to build pillars (that didn't involve sex) on which to support the relationship.

Are there concrete lessons you can glean from these women's views of their relationships? Yes, if more intimacy is what you are after. Whether single, separated, married, or divorced, these women, like millions of others, want to feel connected to their partners. And today that kind of connection necessarily involves men giving more of themselves than they may be used to. It doesn't mean a man must give up his autonomy or that he must be subservient to his female partner. Nor does it mean that he must talk with her every night into the wee hours about his feelings. It does involve expanding the boundaries of what he talks about, what he shares, and when.

Barbara DeAngelis, Ph.D., a Los Angeles–based psychotherapist, cites an example, in her practice and in periodic relationship seminars she holds, of a typical couple *trying* to communicate instead of succeeding at it:

> **SHE:** Let's talk.
> **HE:** What do you want to talk about?
> **SHE:** About us.
> **HE:** What *about* us?[5]

"And now you're in a fight," DeAngelis says. "So women need to give men an agenda. Men like specifics; their brains work differently than ours." Beyond these generalizations, DeAngelis is talking about evolution—not revolution—between the sexes.

Today's men are being asked to "give" things to their wives that their fathers or grandfathers may not have given theirs. And even if they did, it wasn't couched in an outright expectation or demand. In the sweep of a decade or two, men have been asked to develop relationship skills—and they are skills—that may feel totally foreign to them. Is this fair? Maybe. There's no secret answer to this dilemma in the pages of DeAngelis's *Secrets About Men Every Woman Should Know*. There is, though, a logical path to follow. Men can, and should, ask their partners for more specifics. Does she want you to do more, or less, for her than you do financially? Psychologically? Do you ask her about herself often? Does she mind playing the nurturing role (if indeed she's taken that on)? Are her needs for independence being met? Her sexual needs? Are yours?

There's nothing wrong with asking. And even, at times, demanding. There's nothing wrong with admitting it feels strange to tell a woman you're afraid she'll think less of you if you act a certain way (or fail to). By admitting to what feels like weakness, a man can bring his fears out of hiding and take responsibility for them and how they relate to his partner. In doing so he can help make a relationship stronger.

THE START OF THE DEAL

En route to achieving intimacy in marriage, husband and wife often act (perhaps unwittingly) as partners in a deal. If they're lucky, their deal pays off in psychological profit, but the deal isn't easily struck. Because people get together for so many different reasons, they may know *this* woman or *that* man is *the* one without realizing which of their needs their partner actually fulfills. If this happens, partners will at times find themselves at odds, and they may fear their marriage is in peril. In reality, though, it may be merely that *their deal has changed*. An example:

> **HE:** I may need "intimacy," but I depend on my wife (or lover) to bring it out of me.
> **SHE:** I need intimacy, but he won't share it with me. I have to constantly try to force it out of him.

Viewed one way, a deal has been struck that allows for intimate partnership. They both need it (he, reluctantly), but she's in charge of it. Yet viewed another way, the woman in this example may wield more power than she knows. Outwardly, by pressing her mate, she gets closer to him, forcing him to emote, and he in turn gets closer to her. She does the pressing, but the deal seems to work. Inwardly, though—and here's where it gets tricky—she actually may be trying to push her way *out* of the relationship a little, under the guise of intimacy. In some instances she may be locked into the deal and "reward" without really wanting to get at the heart and soul of her partner.

Lynette E., forty-seven and once divorced, has heard all this before. She doesn't think much of the newfangled theories about modern men in relationships. "I think," she says, "you can't teach an old dog new tricks. I personally don't think you can teach a man intimacy either.

"I think a lot of men have feared intimacy since childhood," she adds. Even, I wondered, the ones who are part of the modern sensitive-man movement? "That's bullshit," she says. "Bullshit. I don't think men are any more sensitive than they were ten years ago. I just think they've gotten more clever in how they package themselves."

Curiously, women have also sought better "packaging" in recent years. We saw that in Chapter 3, in regard to the fitness and exercise options that women have taken to in droves. And we saw it again in Chapter 5, in terms of the psychosexual satisfaction many rightfully are seeking today. The difference between the sexes here may be in who's doing what for whom. In recent years women have opened up more than men in terms of self-development and self-help, psychologists say. Meanwhile men are just beginning to hear some of the stirrings that the feminist movement brought to the forefront of women's lives twenty years ago.

A WOMAN WHO THINKS MEN MOVE TOO FAST—EMOTIONALLY: LINDA S.

"I'm a single woman with a steady boyfriend," says Linda S., thirty-four and formerly married. "It's good, I'm happy. I think."

The reason she says she "thinks" is because Linda is still recovering from the psychological hurt she suffered when her marriage broke apart eight years ago. Now she is trying to learn how to give love back in a relationship she wishes she could trust more than she does.

"Since I broke up with Jan," she says, "I have never told a guy, 'I love you.' And I don't think it's hard to feel that. For me it's just hard to say. It might even be the reverse of all that pop psychology that says women think men will run away if women tell them they love them. And it bothers me that I feel pressured by a man—that I have to make 'a decision' already. We've been going out a few months. He says, 'Oh, someday you'll say you love me.' And you know, when you're thirty-four and single, you *want* to be in love. That's the problem with this adult dating." There's more than one problem with adult dating, of course, but in Linda's case the real problem began in her marriage.

"We were best friends, my ex-husband and I," she says, "and I remember my mom saying once, 'When you get married, you lose your best friend.' But I think the biggest mistake people getting married make is thinking that your spouse can be *all* your friends. I think people need to know that their spouses have to have healthy relationships outside of the marriage.

"It's also frustrating for me to hear women who are looking to get married say to me at work, 'Well, at least you *were* married—meaning I've already had what they want and so I'm not allowed to be unhappy about my relationships now. But I think the logic is backward. The reality is, I had a chance at something wonderful and I fucked up."

The hardest part of getting on with her love life after her divorce was that she didn't feel she was allowed to mourn the loss of her marriage. It was "on to the next thing" before she'd thought—or felt—it through. And now, she says, an odd turn of events has occurred. "What I'm finding," says Linda, who grew up in a town not far from Milwaukee, "is that the men I've gone out with are in a bigger rush to get close than I am."

To Linda's surprise, she has assumed the so-called masculine role in the modern adult dating scene, and it isn't quite comfortable for her. At least not yet.

"My perception is that when a guy whips out his baby pictures on a first date"—she pauses, then laughs—"it happened to me about a year ago! I had to think, 'Yeah, *right*.' " Usually, on first dates, it's not the baby pictures women are worried about men trying to whip out.

But the fact remains: Linda is aware she is trying to thwart men's attempts at intimacy even though she enjoys dating them, and she knows this doesn't fit the patterns of male-female relations found in the standard "How to Catch a Man" magazine article. "I think this is a divorce issue," she says, "a *reaction* to it. My experience has been that women my age and older have really been eager to become emotionally intimate much more quickly than I'm willing to."

To give an example, Linda finds it tough to take when a man says to her, on the third or fourth date, "You know, this might work out." She thinks (but doesn't say), "*What* might work out?"

"I've also had a man ask me on a first date, 'What gives you strength in times of stress?' I think that is one of the most intimate questions you could ask someone that soon," she says. "It assumes I trust him or like him enough to tell him—when I just met him an hour ago."

The lesson here is to acknowledge the ranks of women like Linda (there are more of them out there than you might think) and to listen, not look, before you leap. If you do, you may help turn an unsure alliance into a relationship that lasts. This may also keep you from barreling into what might feel to a potential partner like a forced attempt at intimacy. Despite what the women's magazines say, not all women are into up-front intimacy. No more, in fact, than all men are ready to run from it at first brush. Sometimes it helps to forget the stereotypes as you get to know, to really know, your partner.

"Unfortunately love has never worked out for me," Linda says, not out of anger but out of frustration. "The concept of it is fraught with danger. The men have wanted too much too soon, and I can't handle that. I was engaged within three or four months after meeting Jan. It was love at first sight, and we were just too young to really be prepared for marriage."

WHEN TRUST IS ELUSIVE

"I went out with a forty-year-old man last year," Linda says, "who said a wife should be your lover, mentor, friend. Then, at one point, he cried in front of me. I think it may have been a ploy. You know, the sensitive male and all that. All I remember was that he was telling me about his family at the time. What was interesting to me was that *he* initiated the intimacy in our 'relationship' that was all of four weeks old."

Los Angeles therapist Herb Goldberg, who has written often on relationship matters, has a possible explanation for her feelings of resentment and cloaked anger: the actor-reactor process. In this case he would call the crying man the "actor" if the tears weren't sincere. Linda, then, would be the "reactor."

"To the extent that they are reactors, they . . . feel controlled," he says in *The New Male-Female Relationship.* "To the extent that they allow themselves to be controlled, they feel put upon and build up rage. It doesn't matter how 'nicely' they are treated by the man."

For Linda the stabilizing influence of a relationship is trust. She may feel herself falling in love with someone (as she did with her ex-husband), but she will consciously catch herself and pull back if she doesn't trust her partner completely. A woman has to be able to feel secure before she can let go.

"The whole thing about divorce," she says, "is that this huge sacred trust is betrayed. My mother calls it, 'Your loss of innocence.' But you can never recover it once you lose it. Your ego suffers.

"I mean, while Jan and I were separated, I came back from New Mexico to be with him and he had stopped wearing his wedding ring. When we broke up, he said, 'There are six things wrong with our marriage: A, B, C, D, E, and F—and you can't change them. There's nothing we can do.' For years I was pissed off that he didn't even want to try," Linda says. "Then I realized it wasn't in his nature. Or his family's either."

It may have been his problem, or his family's, but the reality is Linda lived with him, married him, and endured a separation from him before they divorced, knowing all the while this repression was part of Jan's very nature. It's not that it should have been her job to "fix it," or even to get her husband to open up and express feelings he had repressed his entire adult life. It was simply a facet of *their* relationship that festered and didn't improve over time. She trusted the bond; her husband didn't. Which didn't by itself make him "bad." But it made them incompatible.

A DIVORCÉE BREAKS THROUGH BARRIERS: DONNA R.

Donna R., a thirty-year-old divorcée from West Virginia, has had troubles in the past with tradition. Traditional families, traditional marriage, traditional ideas about relationships. All that tradition added up to a marriage that splintered a few years ago. But unlike the divorce of Linda S., above, Donna was responsible for the split. The period of rediscovery Donna underwent during the breakup holds lessons for others, especially men. Her divorce had been finalized barely a year before we spoke, but it was still very much on her mind. So were vivid memories of the "model" relationship she saw while she was growing up—that of her parents.

"They coexisted kind of well," Donna says. "without airing their individual grievances. It was an odd dynamic, though. I felt I was protecting my mother. She was afraid to push him to find out what he was about.

"At one point, when my mother wanted to go to law school, my father said, 'No. I'm providing for you, and you should be happy.' That's when I realized they weren't communicating, but I was too young to intercede. He wouldn't let her grow. I thought what they had was ideal, because they never fought, drank, or cheated on each other."

When Donna got married, she realized quickly, though too late, that her parents' marriage *was* her model. And marriage was a dramatic change for her. Part of the reason she was so excited about getting married in the first place was that her fiancé, James, was quite emotional, whereas she was not. "I wanted to experience that," she says. "I remember thinking that to be able to read him so easily was attractive to me. I was so much more on an even keel than he was; there was real energy with that. There was expressiveness."

On the flip side, Donna says, she would never even tell him about a problem she was having until weeks or months after it might have been fixed. Early in the marriage, she was afraid to emote.

"He was my first love," Donna says. "It was on and off for five years, but it was absolutely love at first sight. I found that *very* sensual. He wasn't reserved or stoic. The way he touched every-thing, the way he ate. It was all constant energy. He was the opposite of my father, which was a relief."

Donna fell in love with James when she was twenty, during her junior year abroad in college. He would travel regularly to London on business, which was where she was studying. "We had met when I was seventeen and he was twenty-six," she says.

"You know, he was the only guy I've ever chased, other than my current boyfriend," she says. "Till then I had never been intimate with anyone. I wanted that, but I should have seen the writing on the wall."

Upon reflection, Donna thinks she should have known that her first bond of emotional intimacy with a man might not be the best bond she would ever have. Yet because it was so new to her, she found herself willingly getting more and more involved with the man who was touching her life in an amazingly powerful way.

"I was always playing my cards so close to the chest, keeping men off-balance. Then, when I went to grad school, I realized I had had a sort of 'male' upbringing. I wanted to be tougher than the guys so I'd be accepted by them. In my family only 'sissies' cried." Donna didn't want James to know how vulnerable she felt, how much it hurt to be away from him while she was at school.

One summer before they got married, James and Donna met up overseas, "and he turned out to be a jerk," she says. "I really wanted us to be together and he acted like he never knew me. Then he did the rudest thing I could think of: He acted as if he didn't find me physically attractive."

This devastated Donna—her future husband talking about her looks, her body, her *being*, with disinterest. And eventually it turned out to be a relationship issue, not simply a question of vanity. It spoke to her deep-seated fears and sprang from an unseemly side of her fiancé she'd never before seen. After being apart for a long while—and then finally being together with no expression of exuberance for really being with each other—she felt achingly empty.

"We should have been ecstatic over there," she says. "And what he said to me in bed, about my body and how I looked, sounded like catcalls to me. There was no vulnerability, no real sharing. So I broke it off."

Donna distinctly remembers the details that revealed an absence of the intimacy she and James formerly had felt: "I remember he was physically distant when I was getting undressed. And after being apart for so long, I couldn't accept that, because this was someone I cared about, not someone I just wanted to spend the night with. We sounded like we were saying all kinds of movie lines, straight from a script. . . . At that time he was thirty-two and I was twenty-three, and I knew his family was starting to pressure him to marry me.

"It's funny," Donna says. "There's such a difference now between having intercourse and making love that wasn't there when I was twenty-three. I think they are two different animals—to have a short-term, very physical thing versus a long-term relationship or affair."

About a year after breaking off from James, Donna had a change of heart. "He wrote me a letter, formally apologizing for his behavior the summer before. He said he had been scared at the time and that he didn't know what had been wrong with him. By this time, though, I'd had time to simmer.

"I had a good year of grad school without him," Donna says. "I basically thought I'd like to be friends with him. Through all this James was behaving well. He was still chasing me, so I eventually thought he must have real feelings for me. But I went ahead and had a wild affair with a guy named Roger in April and May [her last months in school]." While Roger was sensual, attentive, and very attractive, he scared Donna off when he told her he loved her.

PREMARITAL CONFLICT AND "RESOLUTION"

This new conflict between emotions and sexual pleasure seemed intractable to Donna. She had two men deeply involved with her, one of whom her parents were steering her toward. The other was a free-spirited lover, who seemed utterly "amazing" to Donna, ethereal even. She graduated, went home to West Virginia, and made a huge mistake. She told James, her longtime beau, she would marry him.

"I had no basis to believe this," Donna says, "but I did think there was something in marriage that would make us better lovers. He was very handsome and, being a slightly older man who traveled a lot, he had had dozens of lovers around the world. I felt this other thing with Roger in the spring was my *first* feeling of sexual power. In a way I was glad I was marrying a man who had more experience than I had. I was relieved. I thought I could show him when I felt scared sexually or that he would know when one of us was 'too busy' trying to please the other person in bed."

To Donna, these were supposed to be the high concepts of sexuality and intimacy in marriage: allowing herself to be vulnerable in bed, trusting her partner absolutely. And she was looking forward to experiencing it.

Others can learn a lesson from the way Donna misjudged the situation and suffered from her too-high expectations. Vulnerability is fine to a point. So is giving oneself over to another. But these "gifts" should derive from a partner's strength, not his or her weakness.

"I thought the whole process would take *ten years* to totally explore each other," she says somewhat cynically now. It's as if she realizes how she brutally ignored the enormity of the sexual feelings she had uncovered during her fling with Roger in graduate school.

"At the same time, sex wasn't a game to me anymore. It wasn't just 'for fun.' I guess I was saving something sexually for James— he was going to be my husband. . . . Then we moved, and he was immediately unhappy in his new work situation. He was not doing well, and I was earning more money than he was. I started feeling guilty for doing well, guilty that I couldn't make him happy. I couldn't distract him.

"A lot of our pattern had been for me to listen to his problems and try to work it out. I'd say to him, 'You're incredibly smart and attractive,' and an hour later he'd feel depressed again. He blamed me for him being out East and for his not doing well. It took me a year to realize this was something deeper than work, that this [marriage] was not going to work itself out. So we separated and we'd talk every three months.

"All this time I would think of Roger, but I also felt I must have been glorifying our short time together because now I was going through tough times alone. I didn't see the lack of a great sex life in my marriage as a problem. I saw it as an effect, not a cause of our troubles.

"When I was with Roger," Donna says, "I think I felt guilty about enjoying sex so much. In the end (after James and I separated), I realized that I was more experienced sexually than my 'experienced' husband. He'd been, like, 'fucking,' as far as I was concerned. He had his numbers, but there was no intimacy. What he thought was wild was location—*where* he did it. But I realized that I was much more comfortable with my body than he was with his. And I felt that was false advertising, in a way, on his part. He couldn't face the fact that I had undergone a dramatic transformation sexually, at twenty-three or twenty-four, before we were married.

"Sex for me was offensive in marriage," Donna says, not in the least defensively. "I was dishonest with myself, rather than letting him know I was lonely, unhappy, and disinterested in sex. By our first anniversary I knew we weren't going to make it." Although Donna doesn't say that the lack of sexual intimacy caused her marriage to dissolve, she is aware it was a major contributing factor.

She and Roger had kept in touch through Christmas cards, and he came back to visit the next spring. "I hadn't started dating yet," Donna says. "But I decided I was going to start again right then and there. It was amazing, considering we had first met and had our affair *three years* before. The next day we were both laughing and saying how unbelievable the sex was, how unbelievable it felt. The closeness, the intimacy, the newness of it, the fun."

Comparing her current relationship with Roger to her marriage, Donna says, "I think we'll go way beyond it. We've already gone way beyond it for so many months. We like each other so much. I remember telling myself at the beginning that it was only physical. It wasn't. It isn't."

The truth is, the physical part of Donna's and Roger's relationship—the good, lusty, rip-the-sheets-off-the-bed sex—laid the foundation for their getting back together years later. They strongly felt that one kind of intimacy might very well lead to another. It's not that they had false hopes at the outset, but they had powerful memories of each other that endured. As it happened, their willingness to be intimate with each other in bed as young lovers enabled them to reach for a higher standard of partnership than they may have otherwise sought. Inside or outside a marriage.

Linda S., the divorcée mentioned earlier in this chapter, says, "To me intimacy in sex is when it feels unforced. It's chemistry. And what I've learned about myself after my divorce is that *I* want to control it more. At the same time, I don't want to think of myself as 'controlling,' because I think that's evil."

For Linda and for many other women, whatever their marital status, this matter of control stirs up a different issue—the "macho" factor. Linda has, over time, come to associate control in a relationship with the male role: He should take control. He should make the moves. He should have the trouble saying, "I love you." What she doesn't know is that in the spring of 1989 two professors writing in the *Journal of Sex and Marital Therapy* found that people who can shed the "macho" or "feminine" roles tend to have better sex. Those who ignore the old notions of what a man or woman should or shouldn't do say they experience more sexual pleasure than those who play out stereotypical gender roles.[6]

"You know," Linda adds, "you really can't rush any of this stuff. You can't enjoy sex until you're ready for it—when you don't have to be talked into it, pressured or threatened. I want to trust someone before I sleep with him. It may even be that you trust their motives, but not necessarily for the next twenty years. It could be just for one night. But if it is, you want to trust that their understanding is your understanding."

THE FALL OF BARRIERS, THE RISE OF COUPLES THERAPY

For better or for worse, for richer and poorer, and for reasons of failed intimacy and others discussed in this chapter, the field of marriage counseling has changed dramatically in the past decade. In some ways it has been swallowed up by the rise of what is now called couples therapy—the same practice with a modern name. According to one man who went through it, the name change to couples therapy is the outgrowth of a recent discovery made by the aging baby-boom generation: "You don't have to be married to want to throttle the person you're living with."[7]

In terms of numbers, the membership of the American Association for Marriage and Family Therapy more than doubled in the 1980s: from 7,500 to 16,000. Meanwhile therapists across the country continue to report more couples among their clientele, suggesting either a rise in actual relationship problems or, more likely, more frequent attempts by men and women to resolve their troubles together.

In terms of success, however, two heads aren't always better than one. No matter what the therapy is called. This is because, couples therapists say, there are *two* sets of problems being aired in one room, so treatment can become complicated. In individual therapy a client and his or her therapist usually agree fairly quickly on the goals of the sessions, even if there are different ways of reaching those goals.

With troubled couples an array of conflicts often arise, with two separate sets of needs that aren't being met. And with an array of problems, a lot of psychological sorting out needs to be done before the therapist and partners can go about resolving them. So even as counselors welcome the increased number of visits by partners, it is too soon to say whether the new breed of couples therapists will succeed where marriage counselors of yore fell frustratingly short.

AFFAIRS AND THE POWER OF SEXUALLY LISTENING

At its simplest, when two becomes three, when one partner ventures into an affair for whatever reason, a previously closed system is breached. At once the original relationship takes on new weight, new pressure, and hurtles into a more complex phase. During or after an affair the longtime partners may have to contend with a severe loss of trust and intimacy and a heightened sense of tension.

Sometimes, though, an affair will lead to startling discoveries about all those concerned: In the wake of new tensions, inexplicable feelings of love and passion may wash over the triangle of the affair (at least temporarily). Of course there may also be a swift downhill slide toward breakup or divorce.

"When I found out Ron had slept with someone else, I screamed, I slammed down the phone, I didn't believe it," says Monica N., thirty-two and single, from St. Paul, Minnesota. "I was crying, and I couldn't believe he actually wanted to hurt me. We'd been together for four years to that point, and he could have had his affair and denied it. But he didn't. I think most men would deny it; most women would deny it if they wanted to keep the relationship going. But he knew me well enough to know it would destroy me if he told me about it, and he did, the next day, to my face."

Monica says that to this day she doesn't fully trust men, in part because of Ron's affair. She isn't even sure that they would have gotten married if he hadn't cheated on her, but the pain is still evident in her voice four years later. "Men and women are different when it comes to this," she says. "There's a double standard. You hear a man say, 'What's the big deal?' But if a woman of his had an affair, he would never stay with her. If he did, it would only be until he found someone he could be with to do it back to her."

Although there was no way Monica was going to consider giving Ron another chance, three of her female friends told her to reconsider. It was as if, she said, they bought into the double standard she so fiercely opposes. In other couples' lives the decision to leave or remain after an affair is often not as clear-cut. For them the line between love and commitment is blurry and dynamic. They may love the other person despite the breach of infidelity and yet not be committed to keeping the relationship intact. Or they may not be in love any longer, yet try to save the marriage out of the commitment they felt when they took their wedding vows. The point is, for better or worse, love and commitment may be seen as *independent*—not interdependent—traits.[8] So, when partners work out their feelings about love, commitment, fidelity, and partnership individually, it may take months or years before they can get together psychologically in order to ultimately decide what to do.

One of the more perplexing questions that arises among experts who study "extramarital" affairs is, Why do some relationships get *stronger* when a triangle is formed? At first thought this wouldn't seem to make sense. Which is why Ethel S. Person, Ph.D., doesn't usually try to answer such questions at first thought. As director of the Psychoanalytic Center at Columbia University in New York, Person believes that affairs are often rooted in unresolved patterns of behavior between partners and their parents—the so-called Oedipal conflicts of childhood.

As Person and other analysts see it, the normal sexual "conflicts" children go through with their opposite-sex parent sometimes leave imprints upon a child. The "competition" a little girl feels, for instance, while "battling" her mother for her father's attention may subconsciously resurface later in life. The little girl, who is now grown up, single, and in an affair, say, may find herself doing battle with a married woman (symbolically her mother) for the affection of the married woman's husband. This would be an affair of the classic triangular shape. And the result of all this mindful jockeying between pairs and triangles, Person says, whether it ends up helping or hurting those involved, is lifelong.

When researchers with the Kinsey Institute at Indiana University measured how frequently couples have affairs, they found and reported in 1990 that 30 to 40 percent of married American men had been "sexually unfaithful to their wives." They have also reported that around 20 percent of married women had at least one incident of sexual intercourse outside their marriage, according to the most extensive Kinsey Institute data on women and affairs (published in 1953!). It's likely that the percentage of women who have had extramarital sex is higher than that today. It just hasn't yet been proven.[9]

"I sometimes wonder how much things have really changed," says Pamela Dunkin, M.D., a psychiatrist in Denver who counsels a number of women in her practice. "I still see that men have most of the emotional power in relationships. I also believe, though, that a lot of women are getting themselves out of that pattern—or at least trying to."

What's interesting about Dunkin's particular view of relationships is that she thinks both women and men know better: They know that the more equal the relationship, the better the chances that both partners will be fulfilled. And while Dunkin believes men hold a lot of this emotional power, she's not sure they've been sufficiently prepared to wield it.

"Perhaps in their own homes," Dunkin says, "dad didn't know how to initiate the warm, nurturing relationship with his son. Now these sons have grown up, and intellectually they know that something different needs to be done."

"We need to change things," echoed Marvin Allen at the First International Men's Conference, "when it's easier for a son to get twenty dollars than it is to get twenty minutes of his father's time." Dunkin agrees with Allen's view that men need to reach out emotionally, not only to their children but to their partners as well. "And they may not be prepared for it," she says, "I think there's something very threatening to men about *really* changing the way things used to be—the traditionally masculine roles of doing the yardwork, maintaining the vehicles, and not opening up to their wives or children."

The final lesson here is not that a man will be able to right a shaky relationship or troubled family by spilling his guts and becoming a selfless, subservient partner. Far from it. What Dunkin and other modern therapists believe is that the opening up can actually be a bit selfish, which is not necessarily a bad thing.

If a man can honestly tell his partner what he wants from her, their children, his career, and his friends, then he can set an agenda of sorts. A psychological one. The reason this isn't seen as selfish is because the agenda is one both partners can work on. And she can, and should, reciprocate with her own agenda.

"I have one friend who has been happily married for twenty-five years," Dunkin says. "And when we talk about relationships, she says the other person's needs have to be just a tiny, tiny bit less important than your own—you still put yourself ultimately first. And this is not your boring, submissive-wife relationship."

Echoing these thoughts in *Intimate Partners*, author Maggie Scarf writes, "When . . . space is provided within the system—space for changing, growing, being different over the course of time—marriage can be the most therapeutic of relationships, the fertile terrain which permits both partners to expand, flourish and attain their full potentials."[10]

In some cases a certain degree of separateness, then, can help right a relationship that's run up against stressful times. Because sometimes you have to become two independent people to solve a problem you face together. There is no way around it: The needs of both partners have to be clear, and clearly stated, before they can truly be fulfilled.

CHAPTER 7

THE PLEASURES OF SEX: INSIDE
STORIES OF AROUSAL AND ORGASM

*The sexual definition of masculinity has changed—to feel like a
good lover today you've got to satisfy your partner.*

—BERNIE ZILBERGELD, PH.D.
"The Sex Life of a Baby Boomer"

*Fucking is more than sex. It's just as magical and mysterious as
talking about God or the nature of the universe.*

—HENRY MILLER
"Reflections on Erotica"

In the minds of millions of women, what makes sex great, what
makes it wonderful, often has little to do with fucking. It is, they
say, much more than that. And sometimes less. Listen to Terri D.,
twenty-six, once engaged but never married, who lives in Los
Angeles.

"I've had two guys who have been amazing," she says, "who
taught me that having sex isn't an exercise, that there's so much
potential. And yet some men look at it as piecework, step-by-
step, then orgasm, then you go to sleep. I mean, when I get in my
moods, I want to stay up all night.

"I want to *play*. I want to work up a sweat. I want to take a
bath. I want to horse around, have fun. I want to spend the whole

weekend with the doors locked—when the most I'll put on is a bathrobe."

Talk about ultimate sexual pleasures seems to come easily to Terri. And as it turns out, one of her all-time sexiest moments had nothing to do with her own orgasm but with a partner's.

"He said I could make him come just by talking to him," she said of a recent lover, "and I didn't believe him. But we were in the car one time talking, driving, and talking very dirty. I gave him about three smooches and he came in his pants. That never happened before. He was embarrassed and upset, so I said, 'That's the sexiest thing I've ever seen. You have no *idea*.' And he was saying, 'I can't believe this, I'm so embarrassed.' It just blew me away. That's the level we were on, literally. That I could kiss him and make him come."

A little while later, Terri explains, the feelings were mutual: "He would touch me and my whole body would electrify. I would break out in a cold sweat—literally. I would start shaking, shuddering, all over my body before we made love. And we did things I know I'll never do with anybody else."

Such as?

"Like experimenting with pain and pleasure. Not blood and whips, of course, but pinching and biting. . . . Then we'd ask each other, 'Does that hurt . . . or does that feel good?' What was amazing about this relationship was that it was so pure in its sex. Because we didn't have the outside influences of, you know, what color to paint the living room. [I had] this elation that nobody could ever touch. And nobody could ever feel. Just wonderful."

THE DESIRE FOR AROUSAL

For a woman a heightened sense of arousal often begins with talking, not touching. Even those women who say their sex lives are good say they wouldn't mind incorporating some more verbal foreplay and afterplay into their lovemaking. Irrespective of intercourse, many women who've thought about it a bit say they'd like their men to flirt with them more. Whether or not they're married. Sure, talk is cheap, but it can also be sexy. If, as author Henry Miller wrote, fucking is more than sex, then by all accounts so is seducing.

Dani C., a single Chicago businesswoman, vividly recalls an incident when she got sexually aroused merely by talking with a partner. "It was when he told me, step-by-step," she says, "what he'd like to do to me. And he used very graphic, but loving, flattering language." But this kind of "aural" sex doesn't take place as often as it might.

Particularly in the 1990s, when so many single adults looking for love are cynical of the dating scene and wary of sexually transmitted diseases, it's common to hear both men and women complain about having to wait-wait-wait before they finally have sex. And then, they find, they may zip through their first-time encounters out of frustration.

In a cover story, "Sex: The New Rules," in *Washingtonian* magazine in early 1992, one D.C. woman said, "My standard now is ten dates before I sleep with somebody. I tell men, 'If you're serious, you'll still be around.' This one guy said, 'Oh, wow,' but he hung around." The magazine said that while ten dates may be stretching things, the "new rules" around our nation's capital appear to be that sexual intercourse is likely to occur between the third and the sixth dates.[1]

It used to be that intercourse was the ultimate act of intimacy. Yet many women today think deep talking is more intimate, more revealing. "Bullshit," some men (and women) might respond. But when you think of it, it really does make sense. Talking, touching, and petting are inherently *sensual* activities, but having intercourse isn't necessarily. When women talk about afterplay they enjoy, they mention hugging, talking, *revealing* things in conversation, and massage. To many women the desire for arousal is firmly rooted in the senses. Fortunately men have complementary desires and analogous senses. We just haven't put them as fully to use in the past as the women in our lives might have liked.

FEMALE ORGASM: FANTASIES AND REALITIES

Obviously women also say they enjoy orgasms. Yet here again, the more you talk with them about the so-called ultimate sexual pleasure, the more enlightened you as a man may become. In any number of ways.

"I was pretty wild in college," says Judy H., twenty-eight, a graduate student from Phoenix. "And I was pretty wild just after that, at twenty-one. But I think I knew a lot about to how to make a man happy—and not a whole lot about how to make myself happy. And I thought I didn't care about that."

Judy's early sexual experiences were a mixed bag. Her fanta-

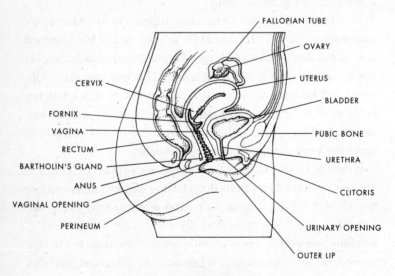

FEMALE PELVIC ORGANS
(side view)

sies were a little about romance, a little about pleasing men, and a lot about "controlling" the hulks who fawned over her. To put it pretty bluntly, she gave a lot of head.

"I was into sex for an ego thing, to see how much I could turn on a guy," Judy says. "It wasn't hard for me. I felt like I knew what I was doing. Except that I thought I was incapable of things like orgasm for myself. I thought, 'Well, you know, it doesn't matter.'"

Judy considers herself "liberated" and feminist, having enjoyed early successes in the workplace and relationship scene before returning to graduate school in 1990. But looking back, she realizes that sexually she didn't reap the benefits of feminism in the late 1960s and early 1970s. She was too young. Her early sex life (in the late 1970s) consisted of a lot of conflicting messages: Go out and get what you want, just like the men. You can say yes, you can say no. Sex is fine, as long as you protect yourself. The

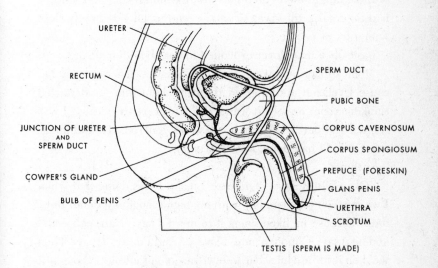

MALE PELVIC ORGANS
(side view)

problem, she now knows, was that her early partners didn't know any more about female orgasm than she did.

Back in 1971, when the writer Norman Mailer found himself the target of messages of feminism and sex, he responded rather mockingly to them: "Women, went the cry, liberate yourselves from the tyranny of the vagina. It is nothing but a flunky to the men," he wrote in *The Prisoner of Sex*.[2] Yet, as is so often the case with Mailer, his literary taunt eventually rang truer than it appeared upon first reading. Twenty years later his words still hold true for too many.

Fortunately, though, not for Judy H. "I didn't realize till much later," she says, "that I could get as much out of sex as a guy could. And the two guys that I've really loved, John and Scott, are the two that taught me about getting pleasure for myself. One [John] was when I was twenty; the other when I was twenty-seven. It's not like I didn't get *any* pleasure before that. But both of them taught me to do things I didn't think I could do. I never had an orgasm till I was twenty, even though I'd already slept with a lot of people."

Basically a male lover explained to her about female orgasms.

"John sort of taught me that," Judy says. "It was mostly because I relaxed and stopped thinking about him—and started thinking about myself. It was great! It was partly because I was relaxed and partly because he was very generous. He did things other people had done, but *differently*."

Such as?

"Okay," Judy says. "Oral sex. I mean I was doing that when I was sixteen [she laughs], with my high school boyfriend. But I did it because he liked doing it to me. I'd say, 'Nah, nah, nah,' and he'd say, 'C'mon, c'mon, I love it.' And I'd say, 'Okay.' Then we'd do it for a while, but I never sort of got into it. I thought it was for him, and when I thought it was enough, I'd say, 'Enough.'

"Then the same went on with the guys from college. A lot of

them liked doing that and I'd say, 'Fine,' and sometimes, you know, I'd act like I was really enjoying it. It's not that I wasn't enjoying it at all. It's just that I never got past the feeling that it was just 'okay.' I guess I just figured I was incapable of orgasm." John was able to change her feelings about oral sex by exploring her genitals carefully and by watching—feeling—her bodily reactions to his motions. And also by spending enough time with her until she felt she could relax completely. For the first time she didn't feel as if she had to rush through it, even though it took a lot longer for her to come than it did for her partner.

Until she found out she could have orgasms during sex (and pretty great ones at that), Judy was satisfied with satisfying the men in her life. "I was twenty when I met John my senior year of college," she says. "I liked sex and I'd been going from one guy to another. It was always really exciting—just to get them off and be with a different person."

When Judy talks of John teaching her how to have an orgasm, she says the discovery was both priceless and slightly embarrassing. She thinks for John it was both gratifying and thrilling: to be able to teach a woman how to have more explosive sexual feeling than she'd ever had.

Halfway across the country, not far from the University of Wisconsin, Madison, campus, Ann M., twenty-two, says, "I lost my virginity when I was fifteen, and it wasn't something I wanted to rush into again. I remember thinking, 'This isn't so great.' At sixteen I still thought, 'There's got to be something to look forward to.'"

Eventually there was. But Ann had to wait until she was twenty-one to find it, with the help of her boyfriend, Kent, twenty-eight. "He's helped me a lot sexually," Ann says, "because he's so open about it. He taught me where my clitoris was."

He taught her *something* . . . as did Judy's ex-lover and as did Terri's at the top of the chapter. So it may be that reports from the sexual front about male wisdom aren't as rare as they used to be. Or at least a lot of men have become a lot more knowledge-able about female orgasm.

"When I first started dating in the 1950s, almost none of my sexual partners seemed to know what or where a clitoris was, let alone find it without fumbling," says Alice W., forty-eight, a married writer from the Midwest. "I even thought maybe I didn't have one or it was in the wrong place. Today men under-stand oral sex on a woman as well as when it's performed on them. I think we [women] are more vocal, *gently* informative, about our desires and turn-on points than we used to be."

Now (at least a minority of) men are teaching some of it to their female partners, while others play willing student. Still, there remains a lot of ignorance about the clitoris, ranging from where *exactly* the clitoris is (just above the urethral opening), to how to pronounce it (accent on the first syllable), to how to stimulate it (that depends on your partner's preference—ask her).

"I think men do know more about women's bodies than they did twenty-five years ago," adds Alice W., with a qualifier. "They may know anatomically more about us from reading, but the actual application in foreplay is still not what it could be."

Similarly, many women wish men would go easier on their nipples. "I think the more experience a man has, the better he is at stimulating a woman," says Joanne, thirty-two and single from the Midwest. "Novices seem to think nipples are turn-on but-tons."

Part of the confusion and frustration stems from what's anatomically hidden. Men may know where the clitoris is, but they may not know that it has roots, and sensitive ones at that, which contain bundles of nerve endings. As medical researcher Josephine Lowndes Sevely says, "[T]he clitoris has deeper struc-tures under the skin. These deeper structures are the organ's two leglike parts that run along the lower part of the pubic bones at either side of the lower vagina between the inner thighs.''[3] When men don't always understand what makes a woman feel good, the clitoral roots may help explain why. Like roots of teeth, they aren't visible, although they can be highly sensitive to the touch.

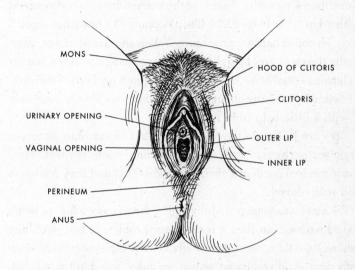

MONS

HOOD OF CLITORIS

CLITORIS

URINARY OPENING

OUTER LIP

VAGINAL OPENING

INNER LIP

PERINEUM

ANUS

ANATOMY OF FEMALE SEXUALITY

At first when Ann M. of Madison learned about what she had been missing, she was more than a little embarrassed. "A *guy* had to tell me this," she says. "I should know these things. But it really helped that he was so patient." She had been sexually active for six years before she enjoyed intercourse, before she found a relationship in which she finally could feel physically comfortable. It was also one in which she could feel "adult," orgasm and all.

Despite the sexual revolution, the myriad lectures about AIDS and prevention, millions of people in their twenties and older (often divorced, with few adult experiences outside of their marriage) have much to learn about sex and their bodies. It matters little that their sexual "equipment" is in prime shape, and this is not anyone's fault, experts say. It's merely a reality.

"At that age," says sex educator Margaret Pepe, Ph.D., of Kent State University, "many of the women are overly concerned with what their bodies look like as opposed to how they work." Judy H. could hardly agree more. When she was that age, even in the throes of great sex, her body-image hang-ups (see Chapter 3) hovered over her. "I was pretty shy about my body," she says. "I definitely was shy about my body." She was able to overcome it with a little help from her friends.

"It's not just what they did," Judy says of her most generous male sex partners, "but how relaxed they made me feel. They made me feel confident about my body. That and they made me feel really loved."

"When I was younger," Judy adds, "it was more a fear of being naked with a man than a body-image problem. I had this thing where I would never take my underwear off—unless it was totally dark. And you know, as you get older, you don't mind that. But then it becomes a fat thing. Like when you go to college. You think, 'Oh, I'm too fat.' " Petite and attractive, Judy has never weighed more than 115 pounds.

"When I'm having sex with someone, I'm aware of where his eyes go when I'm being touched," says Sharon L., thirty-one, once divorced, from Providence, Rhode Island, "and whether or not he wants the lights off. If a man gets up and turns the lights off, I take that to mean he doesn't want to see my body. As sexually confident as I am, it's not the same when it comes to my body. If a man is not responsive, I withdraw. It's that simple.

"I think it's harder being a woman having sex," she adds, "because we're worrying about fat clumps, breast size, fat thighs, stomach 'rolls,' and wrinkles. And then there are some men who make you feel like none of that *matters*.

"You want them to say, 'I love your body' or 'You're beautiful' (even though you can't really ask them to). But if a guy says it just once and then *looks* at you, it can be a real turn-on. I think in our hearts everyone wants to be told she's beautiful."

Nora K., thirty-four and married, living outside of Boston, is another woman who believes the most pleasurable sex tends to happen "when my insecurities about my body are thrown away. A man who says, 'I love your thighs,' is great, even though you know you have fat fuckin' thighs. Or if he says, 'I love your ass—the way your cheeks stick up in the air'—that's when you know he's focusing on you. If the lights are on and he's lookin' at my big butt, I think, 'He must really like me.' If he says, 'You're beautiful,' that's a turn-on for me."

Besides body-image hurdles during sex, many women find they must circumvent some old sex-ed. stumbling blocks in early adulthood. "As far as [sex] education goes," Pepe says, we've come a long way. But unfortunately the questions I hear today from young adults are not so different from the ones of ten years ago."

To gauge the nature of sex and sexual knowledge at that same age, one researcher, Jay Segal, Ph.D., of Temple University, collected some 2,500 sexual autobiographies of college students across the country through the 1970s and early 1980s. He published his findings in *The Sex Lives of College Students*. "Female students who rarely or never achieve orgasm," Segal said, "often cited the length of time needed for stimulation as an important barrier to sexual satisfaction." They were seeking sex, but wound up frustrated. For a number of reasons.

It wasn't that all these young women didn't know how to enjoy sexual stimulation. It may have been more that they didn't feel comfortable enough with their partners, at twenty or so, to talk with them about their preferences. Things like how they liked to be touched; how sensitive their lips, breasts, or clitorises were; or how their bodies responded in sum total. Or it may have been that their male partners didn't spend enough time kissing or caressing them. Or all of the above. Then, too, maybe their male partners didn't have the nerve or wherewithal to ask what more they could do. Sex is tricky at any age, but more so at this one.

"Nonorgasmic females often perceived themselves as being caught in a vicious cycle," said Segal, "which, over time, decreased their chances of sexual enjoyment. Following a nonorgasmic lovemaking session, women often recalled feelings of guilt, shame, and inadequacy."

More clinically, according to Craig Strafford, M.D., obstetrician-gynecologist and president of the Holzer Clinic in Gallipolis, Ohio, a number of things normally happen to a woman when she is sexually and pleasurably aroused. She experiences clitoral engorgement (swelling) and vascular engorgement (more swelling) of the labia; a flush about the chest and neck; sweating; nipple erection; and increased vaginal secretions. When doctors or sexologists talk of "clitoral erection," they are referring to the head of the clitoris and immediate surrounding area, which is composed of erectile tissue. Surrounding this sensitive tissue are genital corpuscles, nerve endings really, which in the right hands (and with the right stimulation) can increase immensely the potential for a woman's pleasure (see illustration on p. 125).

"These are the signs of the passions of youth," Dr. Strafford says, referring to the benchmark listing above, which changes only slightly throughout a woman's fertile years. "Yet many women in their forties will consistently have more satisfying sexual responses than they did at twenty."

"I had my first orgasm at twenty-seven," says Mary J., a single woman living on the East Coast. "Being forty is very different.

When I was in my early twenties, I think I was into the rebellious act of it rather than the pleasure of it."

"I guess at twenty-two I had a list of 'performing' things," says Theo M., twenty-eight, a physical therapist from Cleveland. "Now I don't give a hoot about them. I'll stop during sex and say, 'Wait. It's not about performance now.' It's about having fun.

"You read articles that men like sex this way, or they like that type of body, so you feel as if you have to match up with their imaginary list. I used to do that. Now there's no list. Whatever happens that day happens. And it's more enjoyable in that there's no A, then B, then C. It never gets boring."

UNDERSTANDING HER AROUSAL: WHAT SHE WANTS FROM SEX

If you wished to classify the ABCs of orgasm, however, the best available scheme would still be the four-phase sexual-response cycle developed by Masters and Johnson in the 1960s: excitement, plateau, orgasm, and resolution.

And within that cycle four points about women are often misunderstood by men. First, many men don't realize that during plateau, women undergo what is called an orgasmic platform. It is analogous to a man's erection, in that the soft tissues of the outer vagina swell dramatically, actually shrinking its internal diameter. The now-padded vagina "closes in" tightly on the erect penis, producing pleasurable feelings in both partners.

Second, as orgasm approaches, the clitoris momentarily shrinks out of sight, burrowing back beneath its hood. This may confuse many men, who see it as a sign of sexual turnoff. It isn't. It is actually a further sign of *arousal* late in the plateau stage.

Third, the powerful, ecstasy-inducing contractions of orgasm occur at the same rate in both sexes. Masters and Johnson measured this precisely in their lab and found that the pleasurable sensations surge through the genital regions of men and women at 0.8-second intervals. Why they happen to occur at this predict-able rate is a mystery; that's okay, just enjoy them.

Finally, different from men, women don't require a resting phase during resolution before they can renew the excitement phase. (The "prolonged excitement phase" is not the same thing as women's multiple orgasms, which occur in rapid-fire succes-sion in some but not in all women.) The existence of a prolonged excitement phase means that many woman can be brought to two or three orgasms in a row in much less time than their male partners.

Most people didn't know this thirty years ago, so it is still being debated today. In a recent book, *The Magic of Sex*, author Mir-iam Stoppard, M.D, published detailed charts of the phases of orgasm for both sexes and claimed to show how multiple orgasms are possible for both sexes, and how they differ physiologically. The debates over multiple orgasms won't likely be settled soon, though, for as sexologists often point out in interviews, "There's not a lot of research money available for studying pleasure, much less orgasms."

As this kind of sexual information has filtered through society, so has a concomitant rise in female acceptance of masturbation. Sometimes in big, splashy books about sex and fantasy, such as Nancy Friday's *My Secret Garden* (1973) and her sequel, *Women on Top* (1991); sometimes in movies, like Madonna's "Truth or Dare" (1991), or videos, like the Divinyls' "I Touch Myself" (1991); or sometimes much more privately, such as in one-on-one interviews:

"When a woman touches herself," Grace M., a single twenty-nine-year-old from Minnesota, told me, on the subject of solo pleasure and orgasm, "she knows exactly where to touch. A man doesn't. It has to be clockwise for me, and it has to be just the right pressure."

This doesn't mean, of course, that most or all women prefer to be massaged about the clitoris in clockwise fashion. More to the point, it would help men to know how sensitive their partner is on and immediately around the clitoris. The same way that men cringe at times when their penises get nicked by their partner's teeth during oral sex, women may cringe at forceful rubbing of such a highly sensitive sexual organ.

This is how the editors of *The New Our Bodies, Ourselves: A Book by and for Women* put it: "The clitoris is exquisitely sensitive, and for most of us direct touching or rubbing of the clitoris (especially the glans, or tip) is painful (many men don't know this until we tell them)."[4]

In related reporting about women's pleasure, the authors of *Sexual Happiness for Women: A Practical Approach* say that nearly every woman can reach orgasm through "proper" stimulation of the clitoris—with or without intercourse. This kind of stimulation, the authors add, "is the most common method of masturbation. The clitoris corresponds in some ways to the head of the penis but is even more sensitive."[5]

So what kind of stimulation is "proper"? There is no one answer. However, the best advice a man can get before having sex or masturbating a woman is to start gently—and indirectly. Think of the clitoris not as a button but as a region. Don't rub it right away; rub around it, and don't overlook the inner thighs, the inner and outer lips of the vagina, the skin all over her body, the breasts and nipples, ears and neck, and then think about the clitoris again. Think "gentle," still, for a few minutes longer than you *think* would be enough to arouse your partner. This is what women told me they enjoy when it comes to sex besides intercourse.

"I think the biggest mistake men make," Judy H. says, "is that they touch you as hard as they want you to touch them. And it just doesn't work that way."

"Good sex has so little to do with genitals," says Marie G., twenty-nine, a recently married word processor from Denver. "And I was surprised, going out with men in my late twenties in a hip urban area, how many of them didn't seem to know that touching an unaroused vagina will get you nowhere. It's the wrong place to start during sex."

Then, too, even among men who are "schooled" in the anatomy and function of the female genitalia, women say, they sometimes speed directly there during lovemaking. The most effective time to stimulate a woman clitorally is *after* she has been aroused by other means, such as kissing and fondling. (Remember, there are *two* phases—excitement and plateau—that precede orgasm.)

"Another thing," Marie says, "is that just because there's arousal fluid, that doesn't mean you're ready [for intercourse]. Not at all. It takes so much more than that to be ready for sex, because it's such a high-stress world. At least it takes me a long time to relax. I've got to get rid of the day before I can get into it. I like to be touched all over."

"It's not unusual for men to misperceive what really influences women's sexual drives," says Jennifer Knopf, M.D., director of the sex and marital therapy program at Northwestern. "In general there is too much focus on techniques. What I think needs to be followed up on is the 'relationship atmosphere.' " Simply put, a woman has to be relaxed and comfortable before she can be aroused.

"If a man can say, 'Show me,' or 'Tell me what I should do,' " Sharon L. says, "that's the best, because it lets me know right away he's interested in what I want. But I also think every man should admit up front—at least to himself—that he doesn't know everything about a woman's body, because he can't. Because *every* woman is different."

And yet there is something Sharon and other women will admit to, after talking a long time about sexual technique and what feels good. And again, it isn't all about intercourse. "There is

nothing more exciting than a man trying to learn how to mastur-
bate me," Sharon says. "I guess it takes time, and the more
patience a guy has, the better. Even to be shown how to do it
takes patience and attention. It's incredibly touching; there's
nothing better. And I think that's completely because what's
being conveyed to you then is that you are really wanted—that
he isn't just out for himself. It's like a dance, really, where each
person has steps, and it's a problem if the guy can't dance.

"One thing I'm not sure many men know," she adds, "is that
if a guy is giving you cunnilingus, sometimes he is trying so
hard—and you don't want to discourage him—and this is something I had a real hard time telling a man I used to go out with:
It is much more effective if he tries to cover a much larger area
than just your clitoris. He might be trying so hard—and he should
try *soft*.

"With this too-hard/not-soft-enough thing, you can make the
analogy of someone giving you a gift you're not happy with.
You'd really rather have something else, but you don't want to
exchange it or return it. I mean, people do that: They go and get
exactly what they want. But then I think something is lost; because then it ceases being a 'gift.' "

"There are lots of ways to communicate during sex," Nora K.
says, picking up where Sharon left off. "You can communicate
through your fingertips, for one, or your lips or tongue. When a
man goes down on me, it would help if he knew that a 'hard'
tongue hurts. The clit hurts. I like a very slight touch. I can't tell
my husband this, but I'd like to say, 'Just hold your tongue
there—and let me go up against you.' But if I told him that, it
would shatter him; it's such a fragile thing to say.

"But it's the same thing with men—different men like different
kinds of blow jobs. 'Use your hands,' 'don't use your hands.'
'Hold my balls,' 'don't hold my balls.' It gets back to one of my
main desires: I want to have a feeling of falling and he is going

to catch me. And if I don't trust him, then I can't take the chance, I can't relax. I'll tense up.

"I mean, a woman is a whole body—not just a vagina and breasts," adds Nora. "I can't tell you how much pleasure I get from the right touches to the back of my neck, the small of my back, when my toes are sucked, my fingers, too, my back rubbed. The thing is, it takes the fun out it if I have to tell him this is what I want. The best lovers I don't think need to be told. If you see that a man is operating 'intellectually,' it can be a real turn-on."

SEXUAL POSITIONS—AND POSITIONING

When it comes to intellectualizing the varied positions of sex and intercourse, Nora, like a number of women I talked with, was open-minded yet also a little frustrated. "I want to be made to feel sexy and vulnerable," she said. "I'm usually the controlling one in our relationship, and I would like my husband to lead me through things more."

Nora wishes she could reintroduce a sense of playful danger or risk into her sex life that for one reason or another has dissipated during the past few years of her marriage. The "falling" and the "catching" she speaks of, though, isn't literal (it's not even about danger). It is, however, about trying new positions of intercourse, getting *out* of the bed to have sex, varying the intensity of the petting and mutual masturbation, and having sex—or trying to have sex—that she feels she can escape into. So that she can temporarily leave her job and family pressures aside. The more we talked, the more it became clear that she has, in fact, felt this way about sex in the past, at least with other men.

Speaking about her husband, Nora says, "He is almost afraid to touch me. When he does, it's in a way that's not 'I can't wait to do this!' It's more of, 'Is she gonna like this?' He doesn't do it with conviction. I feel like he makes half-assed attempts to make love, and it doesn't work, or hasn't worked lately.

"I want my man to say, 'This is what I'm going to do to you and you're going to love it!' Or if he doesn't say it, to act as if that's what he's thinking. I mean, I can give myself the same [physical] orgasm. Coming is coming. But it's not the same alone. When I'm with a man, I don't want to be scratched like an itch. I want to be *enveloped*. If I'm not feeling that way, or if I have a sense that I'm not going to feel that way, I'll hold back."

That feeling of envelopment came up more than a few times during interviews. "One thing that I find incredibly exciting during sex," Sharon L. says, "is being manhandled—but not how you might think. Not like rape [fantasies] or abuse. What it means to me isn't brute force—it's a man communicating real raw desire, showing that he really wants you. There's something about feeling his physical power and energy that's a big part of it, that makes it exciting."

Like what, exactly?

"This one man I was with," Sharon says, "when we were really going at it, and he was on top, used to reach around and grab me around my ass with both hands. Then he'd pull me even closer to him—and I tell you, that was a *real* high. It made me feel like I was being focused on and *desired*. But, you know . . . the other fifty percent of it is gentleness, tenderness."

When the subject of positions arose, Sharon was open to experimentation (as many women are), even if she doesn't always initiate the new encounters she hopes to have. Comparing the common, man-on-top, missionary position to rear entry, she says, "I don't think it's impersonal if he enters you from behind, unless that's the only way you ever do it.

"I mean, you want to have the person's face near yours. You can't do that if he's entering you from behind—or when he's down between your legs [with his face]. As a variety thing, it's really great. There's some amazing touching he can do when he's coming from behind." Here, Sharon says, she is talking about having her clitoris or breasts massaged (or both at the same time), while her lover is thrusting inside of her. When this happens with the right man, she says, she is more than willing to forgo that temporary visual lock she likes—looking into his eyes during intercourse and having him return the gaze.

"I can see why some women say it's impersonal," she says of rear-entry intercourse, "because men tend to look away while they're doing it. You don't see their eyes, their expression. Do you *know* what it's like when he looks into your eyes while you're doing it? It's a *connection*. That's what you lose when you're having sex and suddenly you can't see his eyes. . . .

"I mean, I know we all grew up in a culture where it's more natural for the man to 'take' the woman, where women are more often dominated by men—and I admit it's even exciting to be 'taken' by a man sometimes. But it doesn't feel good at all if it feels like humiliation. You don't want to feel like this is *all* that's going on between you."

Oddly there's another instance when feeling good doesn't always feel good: the instance of "forced" simultaneous orgasms. "I remember reading when I was a teenager," Marie G. says, "that sex therapists said you don't need to have simultaneous orgasms. So when I grew up, I wasn't that into them. And now my husband likes to have them. So do I, sometimes, but not all the time. After a while I feel like I can't just *have my own*. I like to enjoy it when he comes; then, when I do. If we always come together—and I guess I should be lucky that we can—I don't know, I guess I don't feel like it's mine. Even though we're both coming, we're coming more or less on his schedule."

Other women mentioned side-by-side positions (both front and rear entry) as being "cuddly" and "softer" than man-on-top intercourse, although they also said what you gain in perceived intimacy you sometimes lose in depth of penetration. While I was aware that the Kinsey Institute estimates that some 39 percent of women have tried anal intercourse at least once,[6] less than a dozen women admitted to me they practiced anal intercourse regularly or occasionally. I surmised that some who have tried it didn't feel comfortable sharing that information with a stranger (me), or else they simply didn't find it satisfying or pleasurable. It is also likely that because of the threat of AIDS transmission and the susceptibility of rectal tissues to tearing or infection, fewer couples are practicing anal sex than perhaps did in the 1970s.

Many a man will say that once he is aroused, sliding his stiff penis slowly, smoothly inside a warm, slippery vagina at the outset of intercourse—no matter what the position—is about as ultimate as things get. Unlike a woman, he has no "hidden" clitoris, no elusive G-spot that requires just the *right* kind of stimulation to trigger an orgasm. (The closest genital analog to a G-spot on men may be the frenulum of the penis, the sensitive band of skin on its underside, just an inch or so below the crown, or mushroomlike cap.)

When excited sexually, the body of a man will typically respond with: a sex flush (coloring) about the chest, neck, and face; nipple erection; swelling of the testes and elevation of the testes closer into the body; and shutting off of valves in the penile artery, which traps blood in the penis and causes his erection.

Further stimulation brings waves of muscular contractions about the prostate gland; constriction of the neck of the bladder and of pelvic muscles; passage of seminal fluid from the prostate, release of sperm from the testes, and ejaculation and orgasm, most often within two to five minutes after penetration in intercourse.

But certainly it's not all about intercourse for men either. Scott R., thirty-seven, a married teacher from Kansas City, says the best sex for him is "when I'm totally lost in the moment, not thinking at all, simply feeling. The only 'bad' sex I've had, though, was still pretty okay." Scott seems to have learned what clinician Paul Pearsall, Ph.D., was writing about back in his 1987 best-seller, *Super Marital Sex*. Based on his study and treatment of more than one thousand couples over a five-year period, Pearsall found that the biggest problem men had with sex was not erectile failure or premature ejaculation but *the failure of men to enjoy sex.*

Pearsall strongly believes that the male-genital focus so long in practice "has seriously jeopardized and compromised" men's potential for true sexual pleasure. In less strident terms, it's as if for years now the women have learned all this *stuff* about themselves, their orgasms, their newfound power and sexual ecstasy, while men have remained for the most part on a kind of static plateau.

As a sex and marital therapist, Pearsall doesn't blame men for this; his work is to help *couples*. "Accused of being selfish," he says, "men are not really selfish enough, for they are too busy trying to do instead of be and experience. Love becomes a product they try to 'make.' "[7]

Jack R., thirty-four, a restaurateur from New York, would likely agree. For he has seen both sides, of women and of himself. "I don't remember much about women having orgasms when I was younger," he says. "Maybe they did—but I wasn't focused on them or their pleasure as much. Now I see them squirming over there in bed and I think, 'That's memorable. That's good.' " Hopefully his partners agree.

"When I was younger, I always thought I'd learn about sex as I went along," says Kent K., twenty-eight, Theo M.'s boyfriend (from earlier in this chapter), from Madison. "I stayed a virgin till my early twenties, so I did a lot of reading about sex instead. And because I was always curious what it would take to please a woman.

"I look back at my sexual experiences in my early twenties, and

I had to consume some alcohol to get my inhibitions down. The first time you have sex with a woman, there is so much anxiety— whether you're doing things right, whether you're touching the right places, whether you can perform. It's like you're performing on stage, even though there's only one person in the audience," Kent says.

"I've become wiser about all this because I've had a patient and open partner to teach me," says Scott R.

As for the "selfishness" question, "It's not that I think women my age have gotten more assertive," Jack says. "I think it's that they have gotten more comfortable saying, 'Would you do this for me?' It's not a demand, and I think it's great if she is relaxed enough to ask me to do something for her that's so private." In acknowledging and reacting positively to a woman's needs, a man can put aside old notions of male dominance and help establish a deeper sexual union. Also, one that may be a lot more fun.

THE U-SPOT: PUTTING THE G-SPOT IN ITS PLACE

When you think of it, without scientific inquiry sex might merely be fun. For years researchers have sought to learn precisely why people feel that they *have* to have sex, or what exactly makes people *love* making love. There are literally thousands of questions about ultimate pleasures and unfortunately not nearly as many answers.

But one of the more intriguing answers to have emerged from the lab recently has to do with the so-called G-spot in the vagina—and what it may be connected to. For two decades now gynecologists and sexologists have debated the existence and location of the Grafenberg spot (named for the German physician, first name Ernst, who discovered it); so far, the debates have brought forth more controversy than valid science.

The G-spot is typically described as a small, sensitive area just behind the front wall of the vagina (the top when a woman is lying on her back), between the pubic bone and the cervix. The trouble in pinning this down precisely lies in the fact that there is so much normal variation between women. The sensitivity of their vaginal walls, nerves, lubrication, and sexual psyches ranges so greatly that the G-spot cannot be considered a supersensitive area for every woman. In addition, its precise size and shape is said to be amorphous; it changes during sexual arousal. (It almost goes without saying that a communicative husband will have more success finding this spot with his wife than an overeager teenage boy will with his new girlfriend.)

The news here is that a new supersensitive area of women's genitalia may soon put the G-spot in its place. It has already been discovered in lab animals, and the crossover to humans is coming (literally). It has been called the U-spot, by some, because it centers on and around, of all places, the urethra, which carries urine from the bladder. Whatever it is finally called, it's an exciting and not yet widely known discovery in the world of sexology.

A few years ago Kevin E. McKenna, Ph.D., an assistant professor of physiology and urology at Northwestern University Medical School, and his colleagues made a surprising finding regarding laboratory rats. They were trying to understand orgasm better, or, in the language of the lab, "the coitus reflex." It turned out they found out as much about female orgasms as they did about males', which they had been studying in the first place.

"We report here," the researchers wrote, "that the coitus reflex can be reliably and repeatedly elicited in both male and female rats by mechanical stimulation of the urethra."[8] The findings were published in 1988 in the journal *Neuroscience Letters*, which is why you may not have heard much recent talk about U-spots in the locker room or in the pages of *Playboy*. It's not as if *Cosmopolitan* got wind of the report and announced it next to some chasmic cleavage on its cover.

In brief, McKenna and his team believe the key to female

climax resides not in the vagina or clitoris but in or around the urethra. They were able to induce orgasm in rats of both sexes by stimulating nerve receptors on the urethra with electronic pulses. And because the sexual anatomy of rats and humans is remarkably similar, the implications for future research into male and female orgasm are likely to be noteworthy. And of course controversial.

But even now, in the early stages of "further research," McKenna and his colleagues believe there may be a *connection* between the U-spot and the elusive G-spot—in both rats and humans. In fact U-spot research may reveal a lot about both the G-spot and orgasm.

"The problem is," McKenna says, "what do you call it? The 'U-spot' was not our term, though I thought it was funny. We're looking at it as a reflex," he adds. "And we know there are neural and mechanical activities that underlie sexual functioning in animals. We still have to prove what they are, though."

If McKenna and his team prove successful in this regard, eventually a lot of excited human animals will eagerly get off on his research.

AN APHRODISIAC UPDATE

In the always stimulating world of aphrodisiac exploration, where sexual "healing" meets chemically induced sexual feeling, researchers recently have come up with a few notable findings. Aphrodisiacs have long gotten a bad rap in serious medical science, mostly because the scientific proof for many supposed sex-boosters has been so sorely lacking. Finally the science is starting to get better.

Sex researchers today are excited about yohimbine, trazadone, and Wellbutrin, three prescription drugs that have been reported to produce sexual enhancement among test subjects. Originally developed for other uses, these drugs cannot be obtained over the counter, and not all doctors will prescribe them for potential sexual uses. That having been said, let's look at them:

Yohimbine, a tree-bark extract from Africa, has produced (experimentally) spinal shivers, pelvic tingles, and reports of more pleasurable sex, researchers say.[9] On the down side, the results reportedly aren't noticeable for two to three weeks. Yohimbine is believed to activate substances already in the body that stimulate pleasure centers of the brain. But, as they say, more research is needed before this tree bark can be considered a certifiable aphrodisiac.

Trazadone, an antidepressant medication, may enhance women's interest in sex, according to clinicians and anecdotal reports. Some women who have taken trazadone have reported that they've had better lovemaking sessions. And other women who were previously anorgasmic have said they believe trazadone has helped them have orgasms. Again, these results are experimental. The drug may actually help women become less inhibited about sex rather than directly stimulate sex centers of the brain. As for contraindications? Trazadone may cause drowsiness or constipation among some users.

Another antidepressant, Wellbutrin is a relatively new drug that has gotten high marks for improving sexual drive among people who have taken it. Researchers at San Diego's Crenshaw Clinic found that in one study nearly two-thirds of the people taking it reported noticeable improvement in their sex lives. Women who had problems achieving orgasm also gave it high marks. The drawbacks? Again, the reported sex effects have taken weeks to develop. And other studies have been less promising. In fact a few years ago before it was released on the market, Wellbutrin was recalled from clinical testing because of reports that it might trigger seizures. (Or were they orgasms?)

WHAT'S MORE THAN SEX . . .

In the end, of course, the joys of arousal, orgasm, and sexual fulfillment aren't really about science. Nor are they about pushing buttons or taking aphrodisiacs or touching a partner this way, then that. Sometimes they're about love, but certainly not always. Most times they are about, well, pleasure. The science, the anatomy, is important, but it's only a beginning.

One of the most significant leaps a man can make in trying to experience what a woman feels sexually is to realize that what he feels through his penis and his loins is *not* what his female partner feels through the walls of her vagina. "I wish men could know, just for a moment, what it feels like for a woman to be penetrated," says Joseph Feldman, a counselor for Planned Parenthood in Phoenix who talks to dozens of women each month about their sex lives, concerns, and contraception. "I think it might help couples a lot."

In fact women may feel very little through the walls of the vagina most of the time, because the nerve cells located along the vaginal walls are not often activated or all that plentiful. (And the clitoris, of course, the nerve center of female pleasure, is located outside the vagina.)

So what may be most pleasurable for a men, the deep, thrusting, in-and-out motions of intercourse, by themselves may provide very little sexual satisfaction for a woman. She may prefer woman-on-top positions, in which she can more carefully direct the pelvic thrusts toward stimulating her clitoris. Or she may prefer more shallow penetration, favoring positions of intercourse in which the tip of his penis rides along the outer edges of the vagina, where the most excitation, nerve response, and swelling naturally occur.

But again, that's anatomy. Besides experimenting with various positions that both partners agree on (side by side, rear entry, seated astride, or anal intercourse, among others), how can men and women get closer during sex? For starters, women say they often fantasize back to their teenage years: when sex was more "dangerous," when anticipation and heavy petting were what mattered. They often speak of "going back to foreplay" and extending (or introducing) afterplay in their adult sex lives.

"I think there was something really great about sex back then," says Judy H., "even though there's a lot that's great about it now. I mean, I still don't think orgasm is it. And I think high school sex is the most exciting thing in the world."

What about noisy versus "silent" sex? "I've been surprised, sometimes," Sharon L. says, "by how loud certain men can be during sex. But it doesn't turn me off. I'd really rather have some expression—and it depends on the guy. I wouldn't want to say what a man should or shouldn't do when it's all about the heat of the moment."

"I *like* to be talked to in bed," says Nora. "The sound of somebody talking to me is so exciting. You can be with someone and you can look, talk, and kiss all at the same time—sound and touch are all coming into it."

Not surprisingly, though, there's dissent from the female ranks: "I don't like shouting, I don't like noise," says Allison, twenty-six, of New York City. "I think a lot of it is acting, and it's really queer. I just don't think it's necessary. It's histrionics, or something like that."

"Good sex," says Alice W., "means lots of day-to-day emotional foreplay. Touching, *quiet* looks across the room, mental moments and understanding. The lovemaking is an extension of all this, and the climax begins building again right after the sex act."

To Alice much of what she considers great sex falls outside the rubric of intercourse. And while she believes that "wham, bam, thank-you-ma'am" thrusting is a good working definition of lousy sex, she doesn't think sex has to last all afternoon. "Good sex," she says, "can also be a quick, wild, wonderful, socko with your mate too!"

"Women want tenderness and affection," says Laura M., thirty-eight, of Baldwin, NY. "They crave it—at least this woman craves it. I want to lie wrapped around a man. A guy's off my list if he can't *hold* me. It was affection that I wanted, not sex. When all they wanted was sex, I'd go home feeling more lonely. Why is that so hard for men to understand? And I think kissing is *so* important," Laura continues, really speaking her mind now. "It's part of making love with someone. I don't like it when you're making love and not kissing."

"The best lover I ever had I met in London even though he was American," Nora says. "We met in a museum in the middle of the day, went to lunch, then went back to his room. He drew a bubblebath; he sponged every part of my body really slowly, he didn't scrub. He washed my hair; dried it; then *brushed it dry*. Very sexy." The way Nora remembers and retells this, she makes it sound as if all the hair follicles in her scalp were erogenous zones unto themselves. In fact they were.

"One of the sexiest things a guy ever did to me was take off my glasses," says Marie. "It was how he did it, and when, that made it so great. I felt like a shy librarian in one of those movies. It was a few years ago, on the couch in my apartment, and I was with this guy I had gone out with a couple times. We were drinking tea and talking, and suddenly as we started kissing, he took my glasses off really slowly and kissed me as he was doing it. I still don't know why, but I *felt* really sexy."

What about kissing different areas of the body?

"Well, people who are *into* kissing my body are the best lovers I've had," Jan says. "Really the best lovers. There should be more of those around."

"I find that before I kiss a guy," Judy says, "if I like the guy a lot, the first night I'm always thinking, 'Please let him be a good kisser.' It's so important. I take it for granted now with Scott. I don't think I ever got serious with someone who couldn't kiss, except in high school."

Judy's ideas about sexual pleasure, like so many women's, have changed with experience and with age. In some cases they've changed markedly (as with her feelings about oral sex). While ten years ago she could hardly imagine why a young man would want to press his face on her vagina and lick her deeply inside for minutes on end, flicking his tongue to and fro between kisses, she now gets quite a kick from it, and then some.

Nowadays, having a lover go down on her is all about her being able to let go, to give herself over to a desire. The same goes for Sharon and for Marie. They've learned to receive extraordinary physical pleasure they used to not even know. All while being reinforced by lovers who enable them to feel they are incredibly desirable, right then, right there, all over. To them there is not much more intimate than that.

For Mary J., though, there is at least one thing more thrilling in bed: "A man who has had oral sex with you while you're on your period—it's not 'lovey.' It's about Wow! It's a mind-fuck, definitely. The biggest."

What some women find sexy about this act is that they realize their partner's commitment to their physical pleasure stretches beyond the so-called conventional boundaries of sex. "I don't know if it's as much a heightened physiological thing as a heightened emotional thing," one woman told me. Depending on whom you talk with, or have oral sex with, it's actually both.

On one level, as a man, when you're having intercourse with a lover, it is perhaps the most intimate thing you can do. You're literally joining yourself with somebody else. And yet what many women say they find incredibly sexy is when you're *not* together and you're still fused—when you're "into" one another enough that you keep this sense of union even when you're not having sex. That's what works for them.

"To me," says Grace M., the twenty-nine-year-old from Minnesota, "the most intimate thing is when a guy comes inside of you. That's wonderful. I think, 'Right now, I have part of a living human being inside my body.' I think of it in a kind of hyperspace.

"I can get sexually aroused in my office the next day thinking about it. I think about having this person's sperm inside of me—and I'll call him and say, 'I was just thinking, we should be together again. . . .'" Long after the arousal, long after the orgasm, a sexual feeling is quite alive. And it's living proof to Grace—to us—that there are times when good sex leaves the physiological world, takes root in the minds of both lovers, and doesn't look back.

CHAPTER 8

HEALTH ISSUES OF

SEX AND

REPRODUCTION

Let's talk about ovulation, flow, and all that other stuff.
—PHIL DONAHUE
"PMS and Men," May 1990

These days a lot of what used to be (quietly) called "women's problems" are mainstream medical concerns. But they are also mainstream media concerns as television talk shows, newspapers, and magazines try continually to demystify women's bodies. The media often fall short, though, in part because all is not equal between the sexes—psychologically or physically. With that in mind and with guidance from everyday women and understanding doctors, this chapter will help put female hormones in context; serve as a short course in why women's bodies do what they do; and explore the ups and downs of a woman's sexual and reproductive health—from the most minor female infection to the most treacherous sexually transmitted disease, AIDS. You can think of it, if you wish, as a guide to some of her innermost parts.

A MAN'S GUIDE TO WOMEN'S HORMONES

To lovers, researchers, and even gynecologists, hormones are the most important but least understood part of a woman's reproductive system. Women and men are often bewildered by their effects, and may at times feel at their mercy. Emotional highs and lows, fertility swings, menstrual woes—all are affected by hormones. And up until a hundred years ago doctors didn't even know hormones existed. Now we at least know these chemical messengers can affect a woman's organs *and* her behavior intermittently and unpredictably.

When it comes to reproduction, though, one thing is well understood: Her hormones jump-start the process. Of course you need heroic-swimming sperm, a ripe egg, and all that. But hormones are the fuel of conception. Female hormones are to thank for a lot of the lusty pleasure derived from sex; they are also to blame for a lot of the pain and discomfort women feel throughout their reproductive cycles. And it all begins in the brain.

Starting from the top, then, the first thing to know about a woman's female hormones is that they are part of her endocrine system. While the *exo*crine glands (such as sweat, mammary) secrete their products (perspiration, milk) directly through ducts, the *endo*crine glands work more mysteriously, more diffusely. The pituitary gland, adrenals, and ovaries—all endocrine glands—use the bloodstream to send their signals to target organs. The four major female hormones are: estrogen, progesterone, follicle-stimulating hormone (FSH), and luteinizing hormone (LH). The ways in which these hormones interact result in fluctuations in a woman's moods, fertility, reproductive abilities, and sexual functioning.

"If I could pick one thing I wish men knew more about, it would be the menstrual cycle," says Holly D., thirty-four, married with two children and living outside Chicago. "It's not just three days of bleeding and that's that." She shakes her head slowly side to side. It seems Holly's husband doesn't understand what exactly afflicts her at various stages of her cycle: the emotional distance she feels premenstrually; her desire, however fleeting, to disconnect from him and from the whole world.

The next thing to know about female hormones is that estrogen is the most powerful. Or to be more precise, *estrogens*, because there are several slightly different ones. If androgens are considered the male hormones (and they are, even though women produce some of them too), then estrogens are the corresponding female hormones. (While the primary source of estrogen production is the ovaries, fatty tissue throughout the body also produces estrogen.)

The known effects of estrogen are wide-ranging and numerous. They include:

- Growth and development of the breasts, uterus, fallopian tubes, and vagina during fetal development and puberty
- Periodic thickening of the lining of the vagina and uterus
- Regulation of the growth of long bones, such as arms and legs
- Development of a woman's body shape and distribution of fat and fatty layers of tissue

There's more, but you get the idea. Now on to progesterone, which is also produced in the ovaries, but unlike estrogen is not produced in the fatty tissue. Chemically progesterone resembles estrogen. It is also found in synthetic form in birth control pills (in the form known as progestin), but the normal effects of progesterone are more limited than those of estrogen. They include:

- Ending the development of breast glands after estrogen has spurred their growth
- Causing the uterine lining to promote development of glands, blood vessels, and different layers within the uterus
- Keeping the uterus from contracting[1]

It's as if estrogen primes a woman's parts to develop while progesterone helps to wind them down. Reproductively speaking, though, things are more complex. While the pituitary gland makes FSH and LH, these in turn stimulate the ovaries to produce estrogen and progesterone. FSH and LH can be thought of, then, as stabilizers and regulators of the reproductive cycle. They prepare and foster the development and release of the egg follicle from the ovaries.

Estrogen. Progesterone. FSH. LSH. A short but potent list of female chemical messengers. Since many *women* remain confounded by the effects of these hormones, their male partners may help bridge some information gaps simply by noting what the hormones do and how they relate to each other.

HORMONES AND PLEASURE

Of course hormones aren't all mysterious chemicals or mere precursors to procreation: They can be potent sources of a woman's sexual pleasure. Testosterone, for instance, which is found in both men and women (though it's more prevalent in men), is often called the libido hormone in clinical circles. Produced by the adrenal glands and the ovaries, a woman's testosterone apparently heightens her sexual enjoyment, although experts can't exactly explain why. This much is known: When women have had an ovary or an adrenal gland removed, they have reported a decline in sexual sensations, interest, and orgasms. Then, too, when women who have reported losses of sexual desire received moderate doses of testosterone, they have reported surges in their sexual urge.

Yet testosterone is not some magical aphrodisiac. The more researchers study it, the more they seem convinced it plays a significant *supporting* role in a woman's sexuality. It's important for her and her partner to know this, should she ever face a decision about gynecological surgery that would involve her adrenal glands or ovaries.

The other notable mystery of sexual pleasure and hormones involves estrogen. When certain women, on occasion and on their doctors' advice, have had pellet implants of estrogens and testosterone inserted in their vaginas, they have noted a corresponding increase in the intensity of orgasm. However, researchers have reported that this effect doesn't kick in when estrogen implants are used without testosterone.[2] Similarly, some women who have hormone deficiencies suffer impaired sexual response, according to Helen Singer Kaplan, M.D., Ph.D., director of the Human Sexuality Program at the New York Hospital–Cornell Medical School.

MENSTRUATION AND MEN

For as long as women have been menstruating, menstrual cycles have been thought of as being monthly and mostly about blood. In reality they are and they aren't. Although the word *menstruation* derives from *mensis*, the Latin word for "month," a normal menstrual cycle for a woman can last anywhere from twenty to thirty-six days, with twenty-eight days as the standard. So *mensis* might be a misnomer. "Period" is actually a more accurate way to describe the regular shedding of the uterine lining at the end of the cycle, approximately once per month during a woman's fertile years. Except, of course, during those months in which she is pregnant or at other times when she is breast-feeding. In extreme instances (such as with excessively trained athletes or anorexics), women may miss periods altogether while not pregnant. If this recurs for months at a time, it is known as amenorrhea and should be reported to a doctor or gynecologist.

If it is difficult for you to imagine what it feels like for a woman to bleed menstrually, remember that it is also difficult for females to grasp—first as prepubescent girls, then as menstruating teenagers. Misinformation and confusion about menstruation can lead to years of psychological pain—or nagging discomfort—about a totally natural bodily process.

Besides blood, a woman's menstrual fluid contains vaginal secretions, mucus, cervical mucus, and endometrial cells that line the walls of the uterus. Most men—and some women—are surprised to learn that the amount of menstrual fluid and tissue released during a period averages only one to two ounces (or about 50 ml.) over three to five days. "It just seems like more," says Dr. Albert George Thomas, an assistant professor of obstetrics and gynecology at Mount Sinai Medical Center in New York City. (The reasons it seems like more range from the occasional staining of underwear to the fact that a woman changes her tampons or menstrual napkins five or more times a day.)

The first two weeks of the menstrual cycle, in which the ovaries prepare an egg to be fertilized, are considered the estrogen phase. The last two weeks, in which an egg is released into a fallopian tube to be fertilized, form the progesterone phase. (These two-week phases refer to an *average* twenty-eight-day menstrual cycle.) As it turns out, menstruation is as much about hormones as it is about blood.

At the midpoint of a woman's cycle—the prime window of opportunity for pregnancy—ovulation occurs. Most of the time ovulation takes place over a forty-eight-hour time span, when one egg follicle has ripened in an ovary to the exclusion of all

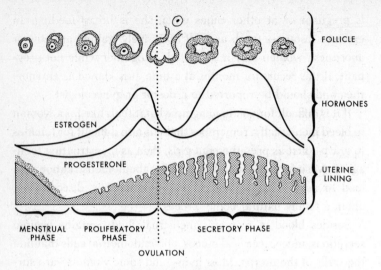

FOLLICLE

HORMONES

ESTROGEN

PROGESTERONE

UTERINE
LINING

MENSTRUAL
PHASE

PROLIFERATORY
PHASE

SECRETORY PHASE

OVULATION

THE MENSTRUAL CYCLE

others. The egg is expelled by the ovary, travels out into the fallopian tube, and heads for the uterus, where it can be fertilized by sperm.

Even before her first menstrual period a young woman has some 300,000 egg follicles stored in her ovaries, from which mature eggs will develop, roughly one each month. Then, at ovulation, the brain shuts off production of one hormone, FSH, and begins producing LH, which is ultimately responsible for boosting the egg out of the ovary. A woman's body temperature may rise half a degree Fahrenheit at this time. Some women feel a small twinge in their abdominal area when ovulation occurs; most don't even notice the moment. A small percentage of women may bleed just a bit at ovulation—doctors call it spotting. But neither ovulation nor spotting is generally painful.

"Also," says Gail Brockman, M.D., a Los Angeles endocrinologist and doctor of internal medicine, "I don't know [how many] men actually know when women ovulate. If they're using the rhythm method of birth control, they should know this. And particularly during a woman's menstrual cycle, men can try to be more tolerant of their partner, because of the changes affecting her."

One other major event occurs at the midpoint of the menstrual cycle. It concerns the cervix, the small noselike protuberance and passageway between the uterus and the vagina. For all but the two days of ovulation in a woman's cycle, a thick concentration of mucus acts as a barrier to protect the cervical opening from any outside organisms. During ovulation this plug turns into a much thinner, watery fluid, saline in nature, that practically *invites* sperm to swim on up inside.

A man who wants to track a partner's changing vaginal secretions during various times of the month can, during foreplay or oral sex, get even closer to that elusive thing called physical intimacy. If, that is, his partner is comfortable with sharing these hormone-induced changes with her male lover. Not all couples find this exercise erotic of course. But it does expand the notion of sexual experimentation.

PREMENSTRUAL SYNDROME (PMS)

For thirty-year-old Sally M. of St. Louis, a pat on the head was what did it. Not long ago she went to see her gynecologist with lingering complaints about premenstrual syndrome, or PMS. Her breasts were swollen and ached, she had "pounding" headaches, felt bloated and fat, and was snapping at her live-in boyfriend. At work she was giving the employees she supervised short shrift. Sally could handle this kind of discomfort for a day or two each month; she thought she should "tough it out." But it turned out she was hurting *five or six* days each month before her menstrual period began. To complicate matters, she didn't feel fully "recovered" until the last day of her five-day periods, which meant she felt the painful influence of her menstrual cycle for up to eleven or twelve days each and every month.

Over the past few years Sally had tried a couple of different therapies: vitamin B_6 capsules and various low-salt, low-sugar, and other nutritional plans. None of them worked. Her PMS was, she felt, inordinately burdensome. Her gynecologist, though, Dr. R., a middle-aged male, told her she might be imagining some of her discomfort. He told her to "try to relax" more. He also suggested she might try to exercise more during the week before she expected her period. She already exercised, though, three or four days each week.

Sally was livid. It wasn't that she expected Dr. R. to employ some miracle cure and "save" her. She merely wanted to talk with him about the latest research about PMS and what he thought she might do to alleviate some of the real pain and irritability she felt. What he told her, she said, amounted to a gratuitous pat on the head. She felt insulted and hurt; she felt belittled. And she has since started getting referrals from friends and co-workers for a new gynecologist. During our last interview Sally told me she had gone to a doctor who had trained at a PMS clinic—a clinic at Mount Sinai Medical Center in New York City specializing in the condition. Sally was hopeful, but not yet convinced she would be, or could be, "cured."

Dr. Gail Brockman, for one, doesn't believe health care providers in general are empathetic enough toward PMS patients. "PMS is believed by women and a few men," she says, "so the didactic physician who likes to have numbers can't measure it. This definitely affects family relationships." For that reason, Brockman adds, "Probably one of my most helpful skills is in *acknowledging* PMS in my patients."

To be sure, not all women suffer from PMS, and of those who do, not all of them suffer symptoms for five, six, or more days each month like Sally does. Nationally 20 to 40 percent of menstruating women report some PMS symptoms from time to time; most sufferers are from twenty-five to forty-five years old.[3] Often PMS hits for only a day or two. (Yet even a single day or two can feel like a lot more.) However long it lasts, PMS normally ends when menstruation begins. According to Theresea Crawford, Ph.D., a San Diego clinician, more than one hundred symptoms of PMS have been recorded in the scientific literature. These include headache, anxiety, depression, moodiness, tender or bloated breasts, acne, nausea, food cravings, sexual cravings, and, perhaps surprisingly, "an urge to clean the house."

Until a cure is found, then, men would do well to get to know the causes and symptoms, and maybe alter your own behavior during the days that PMS hits home. Perhaps you can take over more of the financial or childrearing chores during these days. Or you can give your partner a massage if she finds that soothing. Or, according to Gary Hirmer, director of the PMS and Men Clinic in Minneapolis, you can simply let your partner be alone for a while. That, too, can be caring for her.

Men can also take a cue from gynecologists who urge female sufferers to chart their menstrual cycles and PMS meticulously for a few months in a row. The reason is twofold: to be able to predict certain "down" days (and thus to try to avoid stressful situations); and to enable practitioners to separate true depression, say, from less severe and sporadic depressed moods that have occurred premenstrually.

Terri Hamilton, Ed.D., of the University of California, Fresno, decided to do her doctoral dissertation on the effects of PMS on couples and their coping strategies. For "if I have PMS," she says, "then my husband has PMS." One of the reasons Hamilton was convinced this health topic was worthy of postgraduate study was that "a number of divorces have occurred because of PMS." Hamilton found in her study that not only did couples' communi-

cation fall off during the syndrome, but so did couples' levels of
intimacy and trust.

Hamilton also found that some women had *increased* sex drive
during their bouts with PMS. "Think about it," she says. "These
women are horny, they feel it; yet they hate you; they'll call you
an asshole and confess later that 'I'm a bitch.' " In retrospect
these episodes, she says, were not always laughable. One couple
reported to Hamilton that they actually installed a regulation-
size punching bag in their bedroom to handle such occasional
outbreaks of PMS-inspired behavior. "The label many women
get, that 'She's just a bitch,' " Hamilton says, "is not accurate. It's
not what's happening. And PMS can get worse over time if you
do nothing about it."

In recent years doctors have used hormonal therapy, primarily
progesterone (or synthetic versions of it), to try to smooth out
these rough edges of the cycle. But even this approach, at times
combined with diet modifications and exercise regimens, hasn't
resulted in large-scale success. In mid-1990 the *Journal of the
American Medical Association* published a report that showed
that of 168 women who suffered from PMS, *none* was specifically
helped by taking progesterone.[4] So the controversy (and research) continues because one unfortunate fact remains: As of
the early 1990s there is as yet no federally approved treatment in
the United States for PMS.

"LOVE" HORMONES AND PREGNANCY

By now male "students" of female hormones shouldn't be surprised to learn that hormones trigger a bundle of effects during
a woman's pregnancy. As you'll see in Chapter 10, these range
from retaining water to triggering milk production in the
breasts—to starting the labor process itself. In addition newly
pregnant women soon find that the surge of hormones during
pregnancy may cause them to become nauseated, feel fatigued,

constipated, energetic, sexual, or all of the above.

A few of the lesser-known effects of pregnancy, however, result from substances informally called the pregnancy hormone or the love hormone. Many women have reported feeling more in love, more sensual, more voluptuous during early stages of their pregnancy, and they've attributed this to hormones. In fact the pregnancy hormone—HCG, or human chorionic gonadotropin—switches on soon after a fertilized egg implants itself in the uterus.

The closest substance to an actual "love" hormone is oxytocin, the hormone that triggers labor and orgasm. It is also responsible for some women having orgasms unexpectedly while breast-feeding their babies. (Which can be quite a shock to a woman who isn't prepared for it.) Then, too, the tingling, sensual feelings that sometimes flood a new mother's body while she nurses her baby may spur odd feelings of guilt. While she may have no interest yet in resuming sex with her husband (whether or not she is still healing from the delivery), she may wonder why she is getting sexually aroused from a baby suckling at her nipple. She may feel embarrassed, even, to acknowledge these feelings to her partner.

One hormonal postscript is in order here: Oxytocin also encourages the letdown of mother's milk from the breast as the baby is nursing. So while it may not be nearly as romantic to refer to oxytocin as "the newborn's nutritional hormone," it happens to be that too.

MENOPAUSE AND THE "MENO BOOM"

Looking to explain more fully the world of women's hormones, health professionals with foresight could see it coming: The baby boom that has dominated demographic trends of the United States since the 1950s was at it again. Only this time it wasn't about antiwar protests or relentless rock-and-roll oldies on radio. Instead it was about menopause, the climacteric, the fall-off of hormones in middle-aged women. It was and is about 30 million baby-boom women over the next two decades going through it. And it's about nothing less than this country's first real "Meno Boom."

In brief, menopause refers to the cessation of monthly periods and the end of a woman's reproductive years. The climacteric refers to the entire range of a woman's hormone slowdown. Menopause begins gradually, usually in a woman's late forties, as her periods become less heavy and less frequent until finally they stop altogether. Age itself isn't the cause of menopause—the decline of production of female hormones is responsible. As the ovaries shut down over time, ovulation eventually ceases. The levels of estrogen and progesterone are then lower than they ever were in adulthood.

Not all that long ago the average woman didn't even live to the age of menopause. An American born in 1800, for instance, looked forward to an average life span of only forty-eight years. By the early 1900s, even though life expectancy for women had risen to the mid-fifties, many people understandably still associated menopause with imminent death. Today women commonly live thirty years or more after menopause, as life expectancy for women approaches eighty years. Menopause is now a *mid*-life, not end-of-life, event, occurring at an average age of fifty-one, though women as young as forty and as old as sixty-four commonly report the beginnings of menopause. Mostly it involves the cessation of estrogen production, which leads to the notorious hot flashes, vaginal dryness, potential osteoporosis (thinning of the bones), and other significant changes.

Dr. Brockman, whose wide-ranging medical practice serves women in and around Los Angeles, emphasizes in an interview that menopause is the *biggest* hormonal change in the body for a woman. And, as such, it shouldn't be downplayed by her physician or her male partner. There are a couple of things men need to know about menopause and women, Brockman says. (She adds, though, that not *all* of these affect all women.) The list includes:

- Vaginal dryness
- Subtle depressive symptoms
- Aging, drying effects of the skin
- Hirsuitism (excess hair growth)
- Feelings of unattractiveness; body-image changes are "enormous" (Brockman's word)
- A slight redistribution of weight
- Pain in the joints
- Changes in libido

Some women need to know these things, too, because they may not understand what is happening to their bodies any better than the average man does. Overall, though, there is good news to report about modern menopausal treatment. As the nation's first menopausal clinics have begun to dot the landscape of urban areas (including the Climacteric Clinic, Gainesville, Florida, and one at the University of California at San Diego), more care givers now offer earlier, more effective regimens for menopause than were available before. By focusing health care on the "perimenopausal" years, before menopause actually occurs, doctors and researchers have been able to make this change of life less disruptive for a wide variety of women.[5]

As Brockman explains, certain triggers of menopause (prehormones, she calls them) can now be identified two or three years before the change of life actually occurs. By consulting with a physician and using these predictors, a woman can do a lot to make this often-challenging phase of life less disruptive, more healthful, and more satisfying. For instance, if she chooses hormone replacement therapy (HRT) to alleviate night sweats and sleeplessness that sometimes accompany recurrent hot flashes, she will be able to introduce the synthetic hormones into her body more gradually and with more precision than was typically the case in the past.

Those hot flashes, the wavelike sensations that course through a woman's body during menopause, usually begin in the trunk or chest, then move upward through the head, arms, and legs. Her face may redden, and afterward she may begin to sweat. Some women experience them once a week or less, other women can't sleep through the night; still others feel disabled at work or home during repeated hot flashes. Gradually, over six to twelve months, the flashes tend to subside as hormone levels wane and the body adjusts to its new equilibrium.

Doctors and others who've been through it remind women that menopause is a condition and not a disease. It is a *change* of life, not the end of it. Similarly, the climacteric signals a change in a woman's sex life, not the end of it. Thus, while gynecologists may warn their patients of associated vaginal dryness and occasional pain during menopausal intercourse, they also tell women that if they continue to have sex before and during menopause, it may lessen the severity or degree or number of postmenopausal problems. Doctors also prescribe vaginal creams that contain hormones to help restore and replenish lost moisture.

One fifty-eight-year-old mother of two from Chicago, in an interview for this book, reported that trial and error eventually led her to better postmenopausal sex. It seems the hormonal cream she had been prescribed by her (male) gynecologist wasn't working all that well. After she repeatedly used a plunger-type device (according to instructions) to force the cream deep into her vagina, she realized that it wasn't helping during intercourse. The friction of her partner's penis on her labia and in the outermost third of her now-dryer vagina during intercourse "hurt like hell," she said. That is, until one morning when she tried massaging a small portion of the hormone cream onto her vaginal lips and barely into the orifice, then let her partner's penis "do the work" of spreading the cream into and throughout the rest of her vagina.

Women and men may wonder what the "official" position is on the subject of treating menopause. Perhaps not surprisingly, there isn't one. The Washington, D.C.–based American College of Obstetrics and Gynecology (ACOG) doesn't have a position paper on menopausal treatment, mostly because of its highly individual characteristics. But a spokesman for ACOG says the subject will surely arise at the group's annual conventions throughout the 1990s.

REPRODUCTIVE AND SEXUAL HEALTH CONCERNS

At the height of sexual arousal, when a man and woman are locked together in naked embrace, gynecological health is just about the last thing they want to think about. But think again. For the complexity of a woman's reproductive system demands more attention and closer vigilance than a man's, and the pleasure a woman derives from sex is directly related to her sexual health.

Patrica J., thirty, a pilot from Denver who has never been married, thinks men need to understand female hormones and sexual health because there are times when "women feel more vulnerable than men during sex. Like at puberty or during pregnancy," she says, "due to their hormones. Sometimes [women] feel out of control—and the duration of these feelings is different with each woman."

As far as a woman's reproductive-system "maintenance" is concerned, there are at least fourteen things a man may want to know about. The most relevant are presented here:

1. CYSTITIS AND URINARY TRACT INFECTIONS

The last time Eleanor S., thirty-four, felt her body had broken down was when "it hurt like hell" in the middle of having intercourse. Why? She had a urinary tract infection at the time.

"You get bladder infections from fucking too much," she says, and you know, she has a point. "It's excruciating until you get the medication, so you may end up suffering in silence." Cystitis, or inflammation of the bladder, is usually caused by bacteria that make their way from the vagina to the urethra just above it (the "outside" of the urinary tract) and then to the bladder itself. It may resemble urethritis, or inflammation of the urethra, in that both infections cause pain, although the pain differs. With cystitis a woman may feel a burning, stinging sensation when urinating that intensifies as she finishes. With urethritis the pain is normally less severe and occurs *during* urination. Other symptoms include frequent urges to urinate, abdominal pain, and blood in the urine.

Cystitis can be caused or flare up due to bacteria that have migrated from around the anus, by too-frequent vaginal douching, by repeated, rigorous intercourse ("honeymoon cystitis"), or even by nylon panty hose or skintight jeans. This infection occurs more often in women than men basically because the urethra in women is much shorter than in men (less protective) and because its opening is closer to bacterial sources than is the urethra of the penis. A normal course of treatment begins at home with drinking a lot of water and fluids, especially cranberry juice, and wearing cotton underwear to reduce the chances of bacteria spreading. Doctors frequently prescribe antibiotics for stubborn cases and remind women always to wipe from front to back after going to the bathroom.

In Eleanor's case she was doubly frustrated by the infection because it kept recurring and because she didn't want to "spoil the moment" by telling her husband how much it hurt to have sex with him. She also knows, though, that the infection is nothing for her to feel guilty about. In the future, when her urinary tract again acts up, they'll simply have to put intercourse aside for a time, make it more gentle, or be more creative in bed.

2. THE PAP SMEAR, OR PAP TEST

At its simplest a Pap smear is a routine, effective screen for cervical cancer or other irregularities. Using a speculum to hold the vagina open, a gynecologist inserts a long, thin cotton swab into the vagina and lightly swabs a few cells from the cervix and prepares them for a later look under a microscope. A Pap smear is one of the procedures done in a normal pelvic exam, but may also be called for if a woman complains of pain or infection somewhere in the reproductive tract.

Besides aiding in the detection of cervical cancer or sexually transmitted diseases, Pap tests may also show evidence of a low estrogen level or some types of vaginal-genital infection. It is one of the most frequently performed procedures in gynecology and, when done correctly, doesn't hurt.

Women under forty are typically tested every year or every other year (depending on their medical history), whereas most women over forty are advised to have a Pap smear at least once a year. Women are also told that they should not be menstruating or have had intercourse for at least twenty-four hours before taking a Pap test because blood and semen interfere with the interpretation of the test results.

3. DOUCHING

In ancient Egypt a treatise discovered around 1550 B.C. described how a woman might rid herself of menstrual disorders by using a douche of wine and garlic. Elsewhere in the Ebers Papyrus, as the document was called, vaginal douches of honey, sweet beer, and fennel were prescribed for chronic female disturbances. Times have indeed changed in the area of vaginal douching.

Today doctors and other health care practitioners agree that vaginal douches are rarely necessary for general hygiene and can quite often be harmful to a woman. Women who ask about them are routinely told that a healthy vagina cleanses itself every day and that occasional discharges from the vagina are normal (barring infection). Forcing water and other substances into the vagina may *seem* helpful at times, such as when a woman is concerned about how her vagina smells, yet douches in general are not nearly so helpful as they have been advertised.

Sometimes doctors do recommend douches, usually as part of a treatment or prevention program for infection. Plain warm water, sometimes with a tablespoon of vinegar, is recommended over most of the commercial types. Women should be careful, though, not to force water or air with great pressure into the vagina, because it could affect (or infect) the cervix and uterus.

4. ENDOMETRIOSIS

Endometriosis is at once a painful and a mysterious disease that afflicts millions of women each year. In brief, endometriosis strikes a woman when, without warning, cells from the lining of her uterus begin to grow outside it. These cells may appear on and attach to her ovaries, on structures supporting the uterus, under or behind it, on sidewalls of the pelvis, on the colon, or on the appendix.

Of course these are not changes one can see, and women who may have mild cases of endometriosis may not even notice them. But in full-blown cases women may suffer pain, cramps, abnormal bleeding, or infertility.

With endometriosis, perhaps more so than in other instances of female genital discomfort or infection, there is little a male partner can do to help. It won't lessen her pain, for instance, to massage her or wear a condom during intercourse (in hopes of heightening her chances of recovery without intervention). One thing you can do, though, is to recommend she see a gynecologist trained in using a laparoscope—a device that allows doctors to survey the uterus without having to do surgery.

"We have studies that show this disease affects about 10 percent of the general female population from their teens to about forty-five years of age," says Charles Miller, M.D., head of the reproductive endocrinology and infertility section at Lutheran General Hospital in Chicago. "And if a woman has endometriosis, it doubles her chance of being infertile."[6]

Although doctors don't know what causes the unchecked growth of endometrial tissue, they have various means of controlling it. These include: prescribing birth control pills or medications such as danazol, Lupron, and nafarelin; or, increasingly these days, outpatient laser surgery. Some researchers think the rise in endometriosis is related to delaying pregnancy—having one's first child much later than previous generations of women had typically done.

"We've known for a long time that pregnancy often ends the disease," says Miller, "or at least stops it for a time. [This is] because pregnancy helps normalize a woman's hormonal balance."

5. PID, OR PELVIC INFLAMMATORY DISEASE

When pelvic inflammatory disease (PID) strikes a woman, her partner may not have a clue as to what she is feeling. Lower abdominal pain, chills, nausea, fatigue, vaginal discharge, or combinations of these symptoms may appear. PID may resemble the flu, but they aren't related: PID is an infection of the uterus, fallopian tubes, and the lining of the pelvis that affects 1.5 million women a year in the United States.[7]

In the 1970s, after a sudden influx of PID accompanied the rise in use of the Dalkon Shield intrauterine device, IUDs in general were often implicated as contributing to if not causing PID. Modern IUDs have been tested more rigorously as a result and are much safer (see Chapter 9) than earlier devices. Today most cases of PID are triggered by sexually transmitted diseases, including gonorrhea and chlamydia. And young women with multiple sexual partners appear to be at higher risk—especially those who do not use barrier methods of birth control. Women who use diaphragms, condoms, cervical caps, or sponges, along with spermicides, are at lower risk of PID, although researchers don't yet know exactly how the infection develops. They merely know what has encouraged it.

To discourage PID, during the course of the antibiotic treatment a woman should rest as much as possible and refrain from having intercourse. Besides using condoms regularly, men can help reduce the incidence of PID in their partners by themselves visiting a urologist yearly. Or at least by getting screened for sexually transmitted diseases (such as chlamydia) regularly, since these diseases so often lead to more complicated conditions, like PID in women.

6. UTERINE BLEEDING

One of the reasons men have trouble understanding the nuances of a woman's menstrual bleeding is that we have no frame of reference in these matters: We don't have periods.

Outside the normal patterns of menstrual bleeding covered earlier in the chapter, a woman may on occasion be "spotting," have "breakthrough bleeding," undergo late or heavy menstrual bleeding, or have amenorrhea—cessation of her menstrual period. None of these events is by itself dangerous, but each provides physiological feedback for a woman, her partner, and her doctor.

Spotting generally refers to one or two days of menstruallike bleeding, usually a light amount, that occurs beyond the normal range of one's period. And ovulation itself may be a cause. When estrogen levels drop swiftly or temporarily, this type of mid-cycle bleeding may occur and it usually isn't harmful.

Breakthrough bleeding also occurs between periods, but not necessarily at mid-cycle. A missed birth control pill can cause it; so can starting a new regimen of pills with hormone levels (or a concentration) different from what was previously taken. The bleeding changes color and texture over time, from bright red to brown-red, over the day or two or three of breakthrough bleeding. If a missed pill is the cause, a woman should *not* stop taking the pill. Instead she should take two pills the next day. And she should consult a doctor if the bleeding continues sporadically, say a month on, a month off, then on.

Heavy bleeding may occur if a woman fails to ovulate and the lining of her uterus grows thicker and thicker and finally sloughs off by itself weeks after her scheduled period. The buildup of estrogen in the body may cause late periods as well as heavy ones. Other potential triggers include use of the IUD, PID, birth control pills, or ectopic (tubal) pregnancy.

Amenorrhea refers to a condition when a woman misses her menstrual period. It can be caused by (among other things) sudden weight loss of over ten pounds; having too little body fat; strenuous exercise and prolonged athletic training; stress; or a hormone imbalance. By itself amenorrhea isn't necessarily harmful, but it also happens to be a symptom of infertility. For that reason and others, it shouldn't be ignored.

7. HYSTERECTOMY

The surgical removal of a woman's uterus can be traumatic, lifesaving, or routine; at times it can be all three. Whatever the reason for the operation, hysterectomy is one of the most common surgical procedures performed. An estimated 650,000 women in the United States have hysterectomies each year, and 50 percent of all adult women will have a hysterectomy or oophorectomy (removal of an ovary or ovaries) by the time they reach age sixty-five if the present rates of the surgery continue.[8]

Hysterectomy is considered a lifesaving procedure when performed to remove cancer of the uterus, cervix, vagina, fallopian tubes, or ovaries. As elective surgery, hysterectomy may also be appropriate for some women who suffer from severe endometriosis, pelvic inflammatory disease, fibroid (benign and sometimes bulky) tumors, and excessive bleeding. In any event, while the surgery *may* be commonplace, it should not be taken lightly. A second medical opinion is absolutely justified, and wise. It is, after all, major surgery.

The variations of hysterectomy range from the complete hysterectomy—which involves removal of ovaries, fallopian tubes, the cervix, and the uterus—to the vaginal hysterectomy, in which only the uterus and cervix are removed via the vaginal canal. Today women are more inclined to question their doctor about the need for hysterectomy than they used to be—which is in itself a positive development. There are also new, less-invasive surgical methods available to gynecologists when hysterectomy is necessary. For years female-health advocates have been concerned that far too many women submitted to elective hysterectomy when it wasn't in their best interest—such as for birth control, when tubal ligation would have been safer and much less expensive to perform.

Recently doctors and researchers have also learned more about how hysterectomy can alter one's moods and sex life. For instance, they now know that orgasms may be less intense for some women—or may be much more elusive—after a hysterectomy. In addition, vaginal lubrication and sexual response may diminish if the ovaries are removed; and intercourse may be uncomfortable if the surgery results in scar tissue in or around the vagina. On the other hand, for some women who have suffered for years from endometriosis or heavy bleeding, a hysterectomy in their post-childbirth years may result in their having much less pain and much better sex.

8. VAGINITIS

Vaginitis—a condition and not a disease—refers to drying, itching, and burning sensations in the vagina and vulva caused by a loss of estrogen in the vagina or by pregnancy, douching, birth control pills, or antibiotics. Sometimes stubborn vaginitis may lead to infection or cause undue pain during intercourse. It is at times benign; other times it may force a woman to seek medical help. Those who are afflicted describe the pain as being intense, diffuse, and generalized (unlike what a man might experience if he suffered a sporadic, stinging sensation in his penis as a result of a low-grade infection).

In general, vaginitis infections arise when the chemistry of the vaginal fluids changes markedly. Normally, on a scale of 1 to 14 (below 7 is acidic, above 7 is alkaline) the pH balance of the vagina measures about 4.5, which is somewhat acidic.[9] The pH changes, though, throughout the menstrual cycle and as a result of medications, sex, or exposure to irritants. These alterations set the stage for vaginitis. In addition, when a woman reaches menopause, her estrogen level falls, which in turn causes specific vaginal changes. She will probably notice a falloff in vaginal secretions, which formerly kept the walls soft, moist, and healthy.

In cases of vaginitis related to menopause, a doctor typically will prescribe a hormonal cream that moisturizes and replenishes the vagina, thereby mollifying the painful-intercourse problem. But this doesn't always work. In other cases commercial vaginal lubricants that don't require a prescription will work. Still other cases may require hormone replacement therapy if the condition doesn't respond to milder treatment.

"Sometimes women blame vaginitis on foam spermicides or the jellies or creams they use in diaphragms," says Niels Lauersen, M.D., "but most often what they *think* is vaginitis is really an allergic reaction to the spermicide."[10]

9. VAGINAL YEAST INFECTIONS

Because a woman's vagina is by nature moist and because it secretes moisture daily, early stages of vaginal infections often go unnoticed. Many times it is not until a vaginal discharge appears or an unpleasant smell emanates, that a woman realizes she is infected.

"Any woman who is smart about this won't say to her partner, 'Oh, sweetheart, I have a yeast infection,' and then laugh," says Allison B., twenty-six, of New York City. "I think you should be able to deal with it together."

When all is well in the vagina, it cleanses itself daily by shedding parts of its lining in the form of a clear, thin mucus. By contrast, when a woman is suffering from a vaginal yeast infection, a thick, whitish, cottage-cheeselike substance is present, often accompanied by itching or redness about the labia. The most common cause of this infection is candida, a yeast fungus that usually coexists peaceably in the body. When it multiplies too quickly, or "overgrows," infection occurs.

Pregnant women often contract yeast infections as their hormone levels surge, changing the chemical balance of their vaginas. Other women get yeast infections when they take antibiotics or other medications that may affect their hormone levels. A woman who is infected may also infect her sex partner(s), so they should postpone intercourse during an infection and they should both be treated if symptoms of itching and inflammation appear.

In the "old days," the 1980s and before, women who suffered yeast infections had to visit a gynecologist to get diagnosed and treated. In the early 1990s, the FDA approved over-the-counter sale of the most commonly prescribed antibiotic treatments for yeast infection—miconazole nitrate vaginal cream (Monistat 7) and clotrimazole (Gyne-Lotrimin). These treatments usually work in seven days or less, though stubborn cases take as long as eight weeks to cure. Other antibiotics are available in suppository form, and a doctor may recommend something other than these two medicines. Which is why it is still advised that women see a doctor and not try to self-diagnose vaginal yeast infection at first. It may indeed be a common infection, but it may also signify a deeper, underlying condition.

10. BREAST LUMPS AND BREAST CANCER

Diagnosed in over 135,000 women each year, breast cancer is the most common form of cancer among women in the United States. In addition, more than 40,000 women die from breast cancer each year. That having been said, it should also be noted that at least half of all women occasionally experience some *benign* swelling or lumpiness in the breasts that accompanies menstruation. These benign lumps usually shrink or disappear within the first day or two of the menstrual period.

Because breast tissue is so variable, monthly breast self-exams have long been recommended to all adult women as a means of early detection of breast cancer. A self-exam enables a woman to get to know the intricacies of her breasts and may lead her to see a doctor about an unusual lump or growth if she finds anything. There are two stages to a breast self-exam: inspection and palpation (the touching phase).

In the inspection phase a woman stands before a mirror and looks for swellings, depressions, puckering of the skin, or changes in the nipple, such as discharge or distorted shape.

In the palpation phase a woman lies down, placing a pillow beneath the shoulder and breast she is about to examine. She uses her opposite hand to lightly press and massage the entire breast, working quadrant by quadrant. An important point to note is that the palpation—the touching and pressing—is done with the *flats* of the fingers, opposite the nails, and not with the fingertips. This way she has increased sensitivity and surface-area contact with her fingers, which are in a sense acting as medical instruments during the self-exam. The procedure is then repeated on the opposite breast, noting in both instances where swelling or lumps might regularly appear. (That will provide useful information to a doctor should a follow-up exam ever be needed.) The best time for self-exam, doctors say, is a couple of days after menstruation, before the cycle of swelling breasts and premenstrual changes kicks in again.

For good preventive health women between the ages of twenty-five and forty should have their breasts examined by a doctor at least every three years. Those over forty should have an annual breast exam with a physician, who may recommend an annual or biannual mammogram (a type of breast X ray). Women over fifty should have both an annual exam and an annual mammogram, because two out of every three cases of breast cancer occur in women over age fifty. Among women who have a history of breast cancer in their family, annual mammograms may be advised beginning in their early thirties.

Men concerned about the breast health of their partners may serve as a secondary line of defense against the disease. For example, during extended lovemaking sessions or massages, if you feel a lump in one of your partner's breasts, it is important for you to ask her about what you felt—and suggest a checkup. Yet husbands or partners *shouldn't* pretend to play doctor, examining a woman every few months or so. In this sensitive area it helps to be vigilant, not overbearing.

If a woman is diagnosed with breast cancer today, she has a number of options that weren't available to women a generation ago. Rather than automatically operating to remove an entire

breast in a radical mastectomy, oncologists and surgeons nowadays often perform partial mastectomies, in which a lump and
some surrounding tissue is excised, or lumpectomies, in which
only the cancerous lump is removed from the breast. Lumpectomy, however, is appropriate only for the smallest, noninvasive cancers. It is usually followed up by radiation treatments.

One recent advance in breast cancer screening and treatment
involves a number of "breast health centers" that have sprung up
about the country, usually associated with a medical center or
research hospital. At the New England Medical Center's Breast
Health Center in Boston, for instance, rather than seeing only
one physician, a woman sees a team of doctors and specialists,
from radiation oncologists to plastic surgeons. Dr. Douglas J.
Marchant, a surgeon and professor of obstetrics and gynecology
who founded the center, says it is no accident that the word
cancer is not part of the center's name.

"Women want breast health, not breast disease," Marchant
says, adding that 70 percent of breast problems do turn out to be
benign rather than malignant.[11]

11. TOXIC SHOCK SYNDROME

The shocking thing to some people is that men can get toxic shock
syndrome too, although it is much more likely to strike women.
Toxic shock syndrome is so named because it is a powerful,
overwhelming infection that, unchecked, leads to physiological
shock and occasionally death.

In recent years, especially 1983–85, a rash of cases of toxic
shock were associated with certain brands of high-absorbency
tampons that have since been removed from the marketplace.
Though the incidence of toxic shock is actually quite low (about
10 cases reported per 100,000 menstruating females a year),
many cases that aren't severe may be going unreported.

The symptoms of toxic shock arrive dramatically and suddenly.

They include high fever, blood pressure drop, vomiting, diarrhea, sore throat, sore muscles, and sometimes headache. Massive doses of antibiotics are used to assail the syndrome, and the sooner treatment starts, the better.

Researchers believe the syndrome is caused by a toxin that is produced by staphylococcus, a strain of bacteria normally present in the vagina. The leading theory on toxic shock syndrome postulates that tampons somehow trap certain bacteria and help form a breeding ground for the associated toxins. Doctors, health care officials, and tampon manufacturers all advise women to change their tampons several times a day, i.e., every three hours. As a further protection against toxic shock they recommend that women use tampons that have the minimum absorbency capable of handling their flow during menstruation. They also advise women to alternate tampons with sanitary (menstrual) napkins during their periods. A concise briefing on toxic shock syndrome is printed on foldout flyers that accompany every box of tampons sold in the United States.

12. DRUGS AND ALCOHOL

While drugs and alcohol tend to affect men and women similarly, some of the differences that do exist between the sexes in ingesting these substances are too important to ignore. For instance, the rapid rise of warnings against drinking alcohol during pregnancy is a relatively new phenomenon. As recently as 1973, Drs. David W. Smith and Kenneth L. Jones discovered fetal alcohol syndrome—birth defects associated with alcohol consumption during pregnancy. That discovery in turn led Jones and others to start a registry of drugs, alcohol, and other agents that *may* eventually harm pregnant women or their babies.

"Basically," Dr. Jones, a pediatrician at the University of California at San Diego, has said, "there are all these chemicals floating around in our society . . . that everybody is in contact with, and we don't know what effect they have on an unborn baby."[12] Jones's work has led to the development of teratology, a branch of female-oriented medicine concerned with the study of teratogens, or agents that cause birth defects. What pains Jones to this day is that he now knows prenatal alcohol exposure is "a completely preventable cause of birth defects." Until 1973 women thought it was completely safe to drink alcohol while pregnant.

Going back farther, the authors of *The New Our Bodies, Ourselves* remind us that patent medicines that contained powerful amounts of opiates were routinely sold to women in the 1800s for relief of "female troubles." Today an elusive and vague bias in prescribing drugs to women may still exist, for two-thirds of all legal, mood-altering drugs are prescribed to women.[13]

The point to keep in mind is that up through most of the twentieth century, most research on drugs and alcohol in the United States has been conducted with male subjects. This occurs even though drugs tested only on men may react quite differently in women's bodies, whose biological (and hormonal) differences could well cause unexpected results.[14] Only recently have women's groups and politicians banded together to press for more female-based physiological study.

Women and their partners should make it a point to ask physicians if drugs they have been prescribed may affect females any differently than males, especially when pregnancy is a consideration. Or you might ask how hormonal swings might affect the delivery of a drug through a woman's body. In this regard the time for assuming women's and men's bodies are equal has passed.

13. AGING AND OSTEOPOROSIS

First and foremost, when you think of women and aging, remember that aging is not a condition, illness, or disease. Aging is a normal, biological part of living that happens to be dreaded more than it should be. This is not to diminish the very real age-related changes that occur in a woman's body, such as loss of skin elasticity, menopause, and slightly elevated risk of heart attacks—but rather to put them in better perspective.

The fact is, on the whole, women today are in better shape than generations of women before them. Decades of eating more healthfully and increased focus on exercise have paid off dividends for millions of women in their thirties, forties, and beyond. (Many of these are women who didn't used to think of forty-two as young.) It's not that women today are "younger" than their same-age counterparts of a generation or two ago. It's more that many advances in health, nutrition, and medicine we now take for granted keep women (and men) today from *feeling* the effects of aging as early as people did in previous generations. Jane Fonda's reign as America's video aerobics queen may finally be on the wane, but Fonda, now in her fifties (even putting the question of plastic surgery aside), possesses a cardiovascular and musculoskeletal system that are the envy of scores of twenty-seven-year-olds. Today fifty-two-year-old female bodies that have passed through menopause are *allowed* to look sexy, as the baby boom has aged its way into the "senior boom" of the 1990s.

Besides menopause, other age-related changes of a woman's body include thinning, sagging, wrinkling of the skin; a loss of lean body mass (in the absence of exercise); vaginal dryness; and a thinning of bone tissue that can lead to osteoporosis, the brittle-bone disease. However, women who ingest 1,000 milligrams of calcium daily and who regularly perform weight-bearing aerobic exercise can strengthen bones or stave off decline during the important premenopausal years. And for many postmenopausal women, a doctor may find that hormone replacement therapy keeps bones and joints strong as well as helping with problems of vaginal dryness and hot flashes. Hormone replacement therapy is usually *not* prescribed for women who have had breast or endometrial cancer, who have a history of liver problems, or who have had problems with blood clots.

To some women the psychological changes associated with aging are more important than the physiological ones. And men who understand this can offer support to their partners that, over time, may be more helpful than calcium supplements or synthetic hormones. One recent survey of two thousand people, by psychologist Louise Atcheson of the University of California at San Francisco, found that *60 percent* of the women polled were afraid they would become less sexually appealing as they got older. Only *14 percent* of the men in the survey had the same fear. At the same time *70 percent* of the women were already bothered by facial lines and wrinkles, while only *4 percent* of the men said they were concerned about facial aging. Of course this is just one survey, but men who are aware of its results might think twice the next time they disregard a self-deprecating remark made by their female partner. Her fears of aging may be all too real. And all too frightening.

14. VAGINISMUS

In rare instances, due to an inexplicable fear of sex or past sexual trauma, the muscles around a woman's vagina will literally lock up and spasm when intercourse is attempted. Her legs may lock up too. This is known as vaginismus, and it may result in either painful intercourse or no intercourse, depending on the psychological state of the woman suffering from it. (Note: *Frigidity* refers more generally to an aversion to sexual intercourse.)

Sometimes vaginismus occurs when an attempt is made to insert a tampon or a gynecologist's speculum. It is most often precipitated by fear on a woman's part—anxiety about possible pain she believes will follow insertion. She may have deep-seated fears about becoming pregnant, ignorance about what intercourse entails, or unbridled guilt about sex. But no matter what the cause, the overriding symptom is extreme pain upon penetration.

Women are usually treated for this condition through psychotherapy or sex counseling, and in some cases with a series of graduated dilators, which aid in opening the vagina slowly, step-by-step. With each dilator a woman gets used to relaxing and tightening, relaxing and tightening, her vaginal muscles around it, until the fear and pain eventually fade.

AIDS AND OTHER SEXUALLY TRANSMITTED DISEASES (STDS)

"When I heard Magic Johnson had the AIDS virus," says Sena V., twenty-five, of Chicago, "I got up from my desk at lunch the next day and went to get tested. Any educated person who's having sex today would. And I do practice safe sex."

Not that long ago, before AIDS became known as AIDS, the most harrowing sexually transmitted disease that confounded doctors and clinicians worldwide was known as GRID. Back in 1981 GRID stood for Gay-Related Immune Disorder, so named because in the United States its primary victims were homosexual men who died after their immune systems were rendered nearly useless. In the space of a few years the entire health community of the United States was jarred by a lethal virus that led to the disease that had then and still has no apparent cure. GRID was soon renamed, more accurately, Acquired Immune Deficiency Syndrome (AIDS), as it began to migrate from sections of the gay male population to heterosexuals across the country.

Throughout the early years of this crisis in public health, few people associated AIDS with women because the percentage of women infected was minuscule. Times have changed. At last count the federal Centers for Disease Control (CDC) estimated that 11 percent of all recorded AIDS cases in the United States were women. The proportion is rising; it is not minuscule any-more. And in November 1991, when basketball star Earvin "Magic" Johnson retired from the game after being diagnosed as having HIV, the virus that causes AIDS, he said he contracted it from having heterosexual sex.

In the United States, deaths from AIDS among women aged fifteen to forty-four rose from 18 in 1980 to 1,430 in 1988, accord-ing to the CDC.[15] In addition, AIDS was found to be the leading killer of women of that age in the states of New York and New Jersey. Nationwide more than 50 percent of the women diag-nosed with AIDS in 1988 were black, reports the National Black Women's Health Project in Atlanta.

The CDC and U.S. Public Health Service estimate that as of mid 1992, up to 1.5 million people in the United States were infected with Human Immunodeficiency Virus, or HIV. While people may have HIV for years without having full-fledged AIDS, it's important to note that at this stage of infection they can still pass on the virus to their sexual partners. In addition, the risk of contracting HIV through heterosexual intercourse from an infected partner is higher for women than for men. More than 230,000 fully symptomatic cases of AIDS have been recorded in the United States since 1981. Yet to date only about 5 to 7 percent of the full-blown AIDS cases in the United States have been attributed to heterosexual transmission. The question remains: Will that low heterosexual transmission rate hold?

Yes—and no—according to government health officials. Al-though they don't foresee a heterosexual AIDS "epidemic" in the United States soon, they project bleaker forecasts (and higher HIV-AIDS contraction rates) for people who already have at least one sexually transmitted disease or those who have sex partners who are at risk for AIDS. The complicating factor is that in general STDs have been rising, not falling, of late.[16]

Of the women interviewed and surveyed for this book, AIDS

was the reason most often cited for changes in their sexual behavior throughout the 1980s. Overall these women did not choose total abstinence from premarital sex as a means of prevention; they have instead opted for more careful selection of sex partners and use of safer sex methods.

"I recently bought a friend a designer condom case—rubber included," says Patsy B., a twenty-eight-year-old single woman from Chicago, hardly blushing. "Can you believe it?"

"I used to 'meet' new people," says Sheila J., a thirty-four-year-old single woman, "but now all I date are old friends that I've known in the past."

"There's nothing like that 'masked man,' " says Mara J., forty, a single woman who lives on the East Coast and speaks fondly of her many one-night stands in her past. "But everything's changed because of AIDS. AIDS has buttoned everybody up; it's buttoned *me* up."

In a survey commissioned by *The New York Times* and CBS News in June 1991, over 50 percent of single adults under forty-five years of age said they have changed their sexual behavior to decrease their chances of contracting AIDS.[17]

In interviews for this book, only longtime married or other women who said they were (and are) monogamous told me their sex lives had not changed since the spread of AIDS in the 1980s and early 1990s. And although AIDS is the most harrowing of the sexually transmitted diseases, it is not the only STD that affects women differently than men. The National AIDS Hotline (24 hours) number is: (800) 342-AIDS.

CONDOMS (AND AIDS)

Now that AIDS has had a ten-year history in the United States, various aspects of the disease relating to women have become clearer. Among these important findings are the following: (a) in addition to blood and semen, the AIDS virus (in infected people) can be transmitted through breast milk and vaginal and cervical secretions; (b) these secretions may transmit the virus to a partner through open sores during intercourse or oral sex; (c) menstrual blood can also contain HIV (the precursor virus to AIDS); (d) if a woman has HIV and she becomes pregnant, there is a 30 to 50 percent chance that her baby will be infected during pregnancy or delivery; and (e) women can pick up the AIDS virus through artificial insemination from an infected donor.

The signs of AIDS infection in both sexes include swollen lymph glands, weight loss, tiredness, night sweats, prolonged diarrhea, fever, flulike illness, shortness of breath, and dementia, or mental confusion. In the briefest terms, once the AIDS virus enters the bloodstream, it eventually attacks the body's immune system and, over time, renders it useless. The CDC believes that 25 percent of the people infected with HIV will contract AIDS within five years of their infection. With AIDS the body—operating without its immune-system defenses—is unable to fight off further infection; this is what finally results in AIDS-related pneumonias, cancers, and death.

While nobody knows how many lives have been saved by the public health campaigns for couples to use condoms, there is no question that condoms have slowed the spread of the disease significantly. So has public knowledge that AIDS is passed through body fluids such as blood, semen, and vaginal secretions. But Dr. Robert Hatcher, a professor of gynecology at Emory University in Atlanta, thinks the public literacy level concerning AIDS is high in some areas, abominable in others. And he thinks we, as a society, have barely begun to fight. His contributions in this regard, in helping develop a free condom program called "Condom Sense" at Grady Memorial Hospital in Atlanta, have been nothing short of staggering.

"It's sex education on a massive scale," Hatcher says of "Condom Sense." "We've given away from half a million condoms a year in 1988, to 673,000 in 1989, and 773,000 in 1990 at the Grady Clinic for Reproductive Health [which is affiliated with Emory].

"We provide up to forty color condoms," Hatcher says, "no questions asked." Though there is a survey offered to recipients, of whom the overwhelming majority are women, clinic users aren't required to fill out the survey in order to receive their condoms. The staff of the Grady Clinic hopes first to protect, then to educate, *then* to inquire and collect survey-type data.

Up till now the drug most commonly prescribed to try to slow the onset of AIDS is AZT (otherwise known as zidovudine). A newer drug, DDI, or dideoxy inosine, has also showed promising results in slowing the progression of AIDS in studies in the early 1990s. Until further treatments are discovered, approved, and distributed, however, the bulk of public health efforts to slow the spread of the disease will consist of education, testing, and promoting condom use such as that above. On the research front, by mid-1990, seventy-one medicines and combinations of medicines were being developed by forty-one firms to treat AIDS and related disorders.[18] The seventy-one research projects involved sixty-one different drugs and vaccines, which some AIDS officials found encouraging. Others in the field wish they could be as optimistic.

GONORRHEA

Caused by bacterial infection, gonorrhea has been a public health concern for centuries. An estimated 1 to 2 million new cases are reported each year, and it is thought to be increasing in incidence in urban areas. Gonorrhea may not have immediately apparent symptoms, although many sufferers (in retrospect) remember feeling pain while urinating within two to ten days after becoming infected.

Women may also notice a vaginal discharge, or have a sore throat if the infection was contracted through oral sex. In addition, infected women may note unusually heavy menstrual bleeding, or they may have episodes of bleeding between periods.

Gonorrhea is spread by direct contact with infected mucous membranes in the mouth, throat, and genitals. A doctor diagnoses the disease by taking a smear or culture. If left untreated, gonorrhea can cause skin sores, arthritis, pelvic inflammatory disease in women, or permanent sterility in both women and men. Babies can contract the disease during birth and in some instances can become blind. The primary means of treating gonorrhea is with antibiotics.

Recent reports at the CDC have warned that strains of penicillin- and tetracycline-resistant gonorrhea are now spreading. However, newer, more expensive drugs—including ceftriaxone and spectinomycin—can be used to control the infection in most of those cases.[19] Officially, more than 735,000 cases of gonorrhea were reported last year. The actual number of new cases, though (including those diagnosed by private physicians who don't report all cases to public health officials), is certainly higher than that.

SYPHILIS

This common bacterial infection (more than 130,000 cases are recorded each year) also dates back centuries and, like gonorrhea, is treatable and curable if caught early on. It is passed by sexual contact from genitals to genitals, or mouth to genitals. If not treated, syphilis has four stages. The first sign (and stage) of syphilis, which may appear up to three months after infection, is a chancre sore that is generally painless on the mouth, genitals, or around the rectum. The chancre isn't as noticeable on a woman, though, especially when it appears on the vulva.

Some six weeks later, in the absence of diagnosis and treatment, a fever, rash, and flulike symptoms may follow (in both sexes)—the second stage. Such fevers may subside, then reappear. Or they may completely disappear, although the syphilis, untreated, will not. The third stage, which occurs years later and affects the joints and perhaps the heart, is rarer these days in Westernized countries because of diagnostic advances and antibiotics. The fourth stage, rarer still, occurs when syphilis attacks the brain, crippling intellectual functions. Some doctors say that two hundred years ago syphilis was probably feared as much as AIDS is today.

To diagnose syphilis, doctors use a blood test and a sample of cells from the rash or chancre. Once treated with injections of antibiotics, patients should get annual blood tests for a couple of years, at least, to confirm that the infection has been cured.

CHLAMYDIA

With an estimated 4 million new cases each year, chlamydia is the *most prevalent STD* in the United States today. It is also spread by contact with infected mucous membranes. It is chronic if untreated but also curable with antibiotics.

At first the symptoms of chlamydia mimic those of gonorrhea, but then they may be more elusive and delayed. Within three weeks of infection women may notice painful urination or vaginal discharge and possible urethral itching and abdominal pain, with or without fever. Unlike other STDs however, a high percentage of women may be infected and show no symptoms. Men also often carry it asymptomatically, resulting in a Ping-Ponging of the disease back and forth between partners. But later complications typically follow. (If any symptoms are apparent, see a doctor as soon as possible.)

Untreated chlamydia is a leading cause of pelvic inflammatory disease, which can lead to ectopic pregnancy or sterility. Babies born to women who have chlamydia are at risk for eye infection and pneumonia. Testing for chlamydia used to require a forty-eight-hour waiting period for lab results, but today vaginal secretions can be analyzed in an office visit within thirty to sixty minutes. Still, because chlamydia can and does occur simultaneously with gonorrhea, it sometimes escapes initial diagnosis. A final note: Among sexually active teenagers, the infection rate of chlamydia may be as high as 20 percent.[20] This rate diminishes, though, as teenagers enter young adulthood.

HERPES

Until AIDS arrived in the early 1980s, herpes was *the* scary sexually transmitted disease. It is chronic, like AIDS, but unlike AIDS it does not get progressively worse and cannot kill you. More than 20 million people are likely infected with herpes in the United States. It is caused by the herpes simplex virus, which can enter the body through the skin or mucous membranes of the mouth or genitals. The two types of herpes virus are Type 1, which is typically characterized by cold sores on the lips and mouth; and Type 2, which usually involves sores on the genitals.

For a woman the first sign or symptom of herpes infection is often an itching or tingling sensation of the skin on and around the genitals. Within ten to twenty days of infection, muscle aches, swollen glands, fever, and shooting pains in the abdomen and legs may appear. The trademark sores then quickly follow. While these symptoms may fade without treatment, painful sores usually recur, at unpredictable times. During a first infection, 90 percent of women with herpes have sores on their vagina and cervix.[21] The sores appear on the vaginal lips, clitoris, and perineum, the sensitive skin running from the bottom of the vagina to the anus. (In men blisters most often appear on the penis or in the urethra.)

Although some people with herpes do not have recurrences of the disease, about 75 percent do, with the secondary outbreaks usually less severe than the first. They last from three days to two weeks. Doctors can diagnose herpes by sight or by taking scrapings or tissue cultures from the sores. Pregnant women who have herpes must sometimes deliver their babies by cesarean section to protect the newborn from infection.

Antibiotics are ineffective in killing the virus, but a drug called Acyclovir has proven effective in easing the symptoms. Since this treatment is incomplete, sufferers must restrict sexual intercourse to times when their illness is not "active." A group of people with herpes recently banded together to form support groups to deal collectively with the problems this STD can bring, time and again. A national Herpes/STD hotline has been established for information: 800-227-8922.

GENITAL WARTS (HUMAN PAPILLOMAVIRUS, CONDYLOMA)

Nobody likes to think about warts, much less those found on the sexual organs. But genital warts are highly contagious and may even be more dangerous for women than for men because they may escape detection for long periods of time, especially if they are in the vagina or on the cervix. Genital warts are caused by a virus—human papillomavirus—and, despite their name, they may also appear on the mouth or in the throat.

The biggest threat to women posed by these venereal warts appears to be a possible link they may have with cancer of the cervix. (It was long thought, wrongly, that all genital warts were no more harmful than the simple warts that appeared on one's hands or feet.) The small, fleshy masses tend to grow in moist places, and in women they tend to grow more quickly during pregnancy or when another vaginal infection is present.

Spread by sexual contact, the warts are most contagious at first, then their infectious nature dissipates over time. Treatment can consist of a chemical, podophyllin, which is quite irritating to normal skin, or it may require laser surgery if the warts are stubborn or the woman is pregnant. (In case you are wondering, standard over-the-counter wart-removal compounds often *do* work.) Sometimes, too, the warts disappear by themselves without treatment or medication. In general, though, women who've had genital warts should have more frequent checkups and more frequent Pap smears, as recommended by a gynecologist, to keep a close eye on potential changes of the cervix.

When it comes to the caretaking chores of health care, women have traditionally assumed the lead role in millions of households: from diagnosing and healing themselves to making doctors' appointments or caring for the members of their household. Yet many women claim they didn't volunteer for this role in a relationship or family: They got it by default.

The information presented here can give you some helpful means to balance that inequity. It also gives you insight into what makes your partner feel what she feels. Even if she can't explain all the hows and whys of sexual health, it helps to know a little about the whats.

The Best-known Sexually Transmitted Diseases

	Chlamydia	Gonorrhea	Genital Warts	Herpes	Syphilis	AIDS
NO. OF NEW CASES YEARLY	4 million	1.4 million	1 million	500,000	130,000	45,000
% CASES IN WOMEN	40	40	60	60	40	11
CAUSE	Chlamydia trachomatis, a bacterium that affects mucous membranes in the vagina, urethra, rectum, or rarely in the mouth.	Neisseria gonorrhoeae, a bacterium that infects the vagina, rectum, urethra, or mouth.	Human papillomavirus, a family of viruses that produce skin and genital warts.	Herpes simplex virus types I and II, most contagious when an infected person has an oral or genital outbreak.	Treponema pallidum, transmitted by contact with an open sore during the primary stage of the disease.	HIV virus, which attacks the body's immune system.
SYMPTOMS IN WOMEN	Vaginal discharge, abdominal discomfort, pain during urination, but most women do not have symptoms.	Discomfort when urinating, vaginal discharge, abnormal menses. Often asymptomatic.	Small, painless growths on the genitals and anus which may clump together. May also occur inside the vagina without external symptoms. May be asymptomatic.	Painful blisters on the genitals during the first outbreak, sometimes with a fever and aching muscles. Women with sores on the cervix may be unaware of outbreaks. May be asymptomatic.	In the first stage, reddish-brown sores on the mouth and/or genitals which may disappear, though the bacteria remain; in the second, more infectious stage, a widespread skin rash. May be asymptomatic.	Extreme fatigue, fever, swollen lymph nodes, weight loss, night sweats, susceptibility to other diseases. May be asymptomatic at first.

SYMPTOMS IN MEN	Pain during urination, discharge from penis. May be asymptomatic.	Discharge from the penis, pain during urination. May be asymptomatic.	Painless growths that usually appear on penis but may also appear on urethra or in rectal area. May be asymptomatic.	Blisters anywhere on the genitalia, usually on the penis. May be asymptomatic.	Same as for women.	Same as for women.
WHEN SYMPTOMS APPEAR	1 to 3 weeks after infection.	1 to 30 days after infection.	3 weeks to 8 months after infection.	2 to 20 days after infection.	2 to 6 weeks after infection.	Can be 6 months, but the average period is 11 years after infection.
CONSEQUENCES FOR WOMEN IF UNTREATED	Can cause pelvic inflammatory disease and eventual sterility. Can also cause cystitis, mucopurulent cervicitis.	Can cause pelvic inflammatory disease and eventual sterility. Can also cause arthritis.	May be associated with cervical cancer. In pregnancy, warts may necessitate a cesarean section.	Vaginal outbreak in pregnancy may be a problem.	Paralysis, convulsions, brain damage, and possible death.	Death.
DIAGNOSIS	Culture of secretions.	Culture of secretions from cervix, throat, or rectum; results available within two days.	Visual exam for external warts; Pap test for cervical warts.	Visual examination and viral culture of lesion.	Blood test.	A blood test can detect antibodies indicating virus presence.
TREATMENT	10 to 14 days of tetracycline or erythromycin.	Penicillin, although some new strains are resistant to penicillin and must be treated with other antibiotics.	No known cure. Removal of warts with laser surgery or cryotherapy.	No known cure, but can be controlled with the antiviral drug acyclovir. Women with herpes should have a Pap test at least yearly.	Penicillin or other appropriate antibiotic.	AZT, which inhibits the replication of the HIV virus, has been shown to extend life. DDI and DDC are also now prescribed.

CHAPTER 9

BIRTH CONTROL NEWS AND

WOMEN'S VIEWS

When it comes to contraception, the United States is a Third World Country.

—DAVID GRIMES, M.D.

To millions of men birth control is literally a drag. Sometimes it drags out uncomfortable moments during sex. Other times it drags us into discussions we're not comfortable having. It may be considered a hindrance, even as we acknowledge it is a necessary hindrance. But then, we don't get pregnant. For some couples, though, getting comfortable with contraception isn't so much a drag as it is liberating. When this occurs, birth control can help couples make love without fear, without holding back that little something they may not have realized they were holding back. It can serve as a kind of sexual expression.

With all the modern-day concerns about unintended pregnancy and STDs, conversations about contraceptives have become icebreakers in the bedroom more often than ever. Instead of ignoring the issue of birth control, many men today broach the subject well before entering the bedroom. But no matter what birth control method(s) a couple uses, this form of "sexual expression" is too important for a man to ignore—or to leave completely in the hands of his partner. Especially when you stop to consider that in the United States more than half of all pregnancies today are unintended. (In this chapter, birth control devices are discussed primarily in terms of pregnancy prevention. Sexually transmitted diseases are covered in more detail in Chapter 8.)

THE BIRTH CONTROL PILL

Of all the ways to prevent pregnancy, the birth control pill is the most powerful and effective means short of sterilization. It physically alters a woman's reproductive cycle and suppresses ovulation so that an egg cannot mature as it normally would during a woman's menstrual cycle. No mature egg, no way for it to be fertilized by sperm. When used correctly, the pill has a track record of 97 to 99 percent effectiveness.[1]

The power of the pill is also reflected in the liberating effects it has had on women's sex lives and psyches since its widespread introduction in 1960. Early proponents of the pill felt that if women could control their fertility precisely and predictably, they could concentrate more on their sexual pleasure and less on the fear of pregnancy. So could men, for that matter. And so we both have.

In its first two years of distribution in the United States, 750,000 women tried the pill. Today more than 10.5 million American women use it. For years it has been argued that the pill was the most important cause of the sexual revolution of the

1960s, even though feminist Gloria Steinem, among others, has asserted the revolution was already well under way prior to the widespread availability of the pill.

Debbie M., twenty-five, a graduate student in Boston who was born after the pill was introduced here, says, "I loved the pill, but I stopped using it because I stopped seeing somebody regularly. I didn't have a problem forgetting when to take it or anything. You get into a routine, like taking your vitamins. I had side effects for a few days and that was it. I didn't gain weight, but my breasts got bigger, which was nice."

Liza R., twenty-one, a student in Rhode Island, got a lot of her information about the pill—her method of choice—at her college health services center. When asked why she prefers it, she says, "Because it has the highest success rate with what seems to be the lowest chance of things screwing up." (Liza insists her partner use a condom as well, to protect against sexually transmitted diseases.)

Modern birth control pills, which must be prescribed by physicians, come in twenty-, twenty-one-, or twenty-eight-day packages. Among those the twenty-one-day packs are the most commonly used. (The twenty-eight-day packs include seven days of "no-hormone" pills—placebos—to make the scheduling easier to keep track of.) Typically a woman might start taking the pills on the first Sunday after her last period has started, one pill a day, for twenty-one days. Then no pills (or a placebo) for seven days; and the next pack starts again on Sunday.

If a pill is occasionally missed, a woman can take two the next day to catch up. But if pills are missed three days in a row, the user should stop taking them for the rest of that pill cycle. She should then wait for her period; then start a new pill cycle again *after* her period starts as she had done before the interruption. A further caution: Despite popular belief, the pill does not go to work immediately. For the first three weeks of a pill cycle, a second birth control method should also be used. (Similarly a woman can stop taking the pill at any time—when she finishes a pack or before she's finished it—but there is no protective carryover effect. She and her partner must use another form of birth control immediately.)

What exactly is the pill? When people talk of it nowadays, they are referring to one of at least three kinds of pills prescribed most often. The first, the *combined* contraceptive pill, contains both synthetic estrogens and progestins and is the most popular of the three. The second is a *progestin-only* pill. The third and least common is a *"morning after,"* estrogen-laden pill that is used after birth control accidents or failures, but should not be used regularly in this manner. Hormones are powerful stuff.

Because the concentration of estrogen and other hormones in the combined pill today is much lower than those used in the 1960s and 1970s, the modern version is considered much safer for women to use. The earliest pills brought numerous reports of side effects, such as blood-clotting disorders, mood changes, depression, and weight gain. They also raised questions of increased long-term risk for blood clots, stroke, and cancer. Though pills are indeed safer today, not all of the relevant medical questions about them have been dismissed. For instance, one 1990 study from the Centers for Disease Control showed a potential link with breast cancer under the age of thirty-five among pill users, although the overall rate of breast cancer in those years is still quite low.

On the positive side, today's combined pills offer some protection against ovarian and endometrial cancers. And according to the Alan Guttmacher Institute, a New York–based, nonprofit group that studies reproductive issues, the net effect of taking the pill actually reduces a woman's cancer risks. At the same time many women over forty and those who smoke are strongly cautioned against taking the pill, because of reports of possible links with slightly higher rates of breast cancer and circulatory disorders. Gynecologists can explain these benefits and risks to both partners at the time of an exam or when pills are prescribed.

The second type of pill, the progestin-only pill, is more of a mystery to experts in terms of how exactly it works. But it does, almost as effectively as the combined pill. It is 98.5 to 99 percent effective when used correctly (and no pills are forgotten or skipped). Many women feel safer taking these because they contain no estrogen and offer nearly the same contraceptive protection. The progestin-only pills are taken one per day, continuously, beginning on the first day of a woman's period. These pills are believed to prevent pregnancy primarily in two ways: They help keep the cervical mucus tough and pluglike, acting every day of the month as a barrier to sperm, and they keep the lining of the uterus inhospitable to an egg.

The third type of oral contraceptive, the morning-after pill, is the least familiar and has the highest concentration of estrogen. It offers a woman control over some unplanned, high-risk-of-pregnancy sex acts, such as intercourse without protection, intercourse with condoms that break, diaphragms that slip out of place, incorrect use of contraceptive foams or jellies, or instances of sexual assault or rape.

Taking two Ovrals (a brand of combined pill) the day after unprotected intercourse and taking two more twelve hours later, "is 99 percent effective as a contraceptive," says Dr. Louise Tyrer, a spokeswoman at Planned Parenthood in New York City. This method has not been approved by the FDA for widespread use, but has been in use for years, gynecologists say. And while taking oral contraceptives in this manner is not illegal, doctors and drug companies remain hesitant to *promote* what essentially is an overdose of oral contraceptives. Dr.

George Thomas, of Mount Sinai Medical Center in New York City, says it is an *extreme* birth control measure, but is not normally hazardous to a woman if taken under a doctor's supervision.

When gynecologists explain the pill to women and their partners inquiring about it, they often say that the pill "mimics" pregnancy—that it tricks the body into thinking it is already pregnant. That's partly true, but women who take the pill do continue to have menstrual periods, unlike when they are pregnant. However, these menstrual cycles—known as pill cycles—are controlled by the synthetic hormones of the pill instead of by the endocrine glands and ovaries. And as long as a woman is on the pill, she will not ovulate or, depending on which pill she takes, her ovulation will be suppressed.

Because oral contraceptives in general are so effective in preventing pregnancy when used correctly, some new users have a false sense of security about them and can get careless. Moreover, since the overwhelming majority of pill users today are young, from fifteen to twenty-five years of age, they tend to make a lot of inadvertent mistakes. Sometimes when women miss a pill, or for other unexplained reasons, a kind of miniperiod ensues, called breakthrough bleeding. The estrogen cycle is thrown off temporarily, and a woman may spot, or bleed, for a day or two.

"Breakthrough bleeding is common," says Dr. Thomas of Mount Sinai, "but a woman should know that when this happens, she should not stop taking the pill. That [the missed pill] may be what caused the bleeding in the first place. She should instead take two pills the day after she missed one." If both women and men know this before a woman goes on the pill, they won't mistakenly blame the pill for the spotting.

BIRTH CONTROL BOX SCORE: THE BIRTH CONTROL PILL

PREGNANCY PREVENTION: 97–99 percent effective when used
correctly.

STD PREVENTION: Low; doesn't protect against gonorrhea or
chlamydia; but does thicken cervical mucus, which protects
upper genital tract against pelvic inflammatory disease (PID).

COST: Up to $20 per month, plus doctor visit; less expensive at
university health centers and family-planning clinics.

PRESCRIPTION NEEDED: Yes.

THE CONDOM:

It used to be that a condom was a condom was a condom. You
were told not to keep them in your wallet, but you sometimes did
anyway. You joked about them. They looked silly, they sounded
silly: "latex *sheaths*," "prophy-*lac*-tics." They felt silly. Then,
finally, on various occasions in adolescence or early adulthood
you rolled them over your erect penis during sex and they formed
a barrier kind of birth control. You made sure to leave a pinch of
room at the tip of the condom for your ejaculate and squeezed the
reservoir at the tip to rid it of excess air so that it wouldn't burst.
And after you came, you were careful to hold the base of the
condom tightly as you withdrew from your partner so that it
wouldn't slip off or leak. You did the right things. Maybe you
complained a bit about the loss of sensitivity you felt inside a
woman while wearing a rubber. Or maybe you kept that to
yourself. Times change.

"I want skin on skin," said a young man from the South Side
of Chicago not long ago at a Planned Parenthood group session
for males interested in learning more about sex and sex education. He didn't want to have to use condoms.

When AIDS arrived in the early 1980s, condoms were found to be the most effective protection against the disease short of abstinence (see Chapter 8). For millions of men, skin on skin would have to wait awhile. As the production and sales of condoms boomed, condom design inevitably began to change.

In 1987, while on assignment for a business magazine, Jim Thornton, a married writer in his mid-thirties from Minnesota, observed the making of thousands of newfangled condoms inside the factory of the Minneapolis-based Mentor Corporation. He also witnessed the testing of these condoms under way at a furious rate:

"A metallic penis picks up its pace," Thornton wrote, "dipping with renewed vigor in and out of a well-lubricated orifice." He described the sound produced during this process as a cross between a bubble bursting and the squeaky wail of a squeegee. It didn't sound pleasant. Yet what Thornton observed that day was revolutionary in the long-sleepy market for prophylactics, condoms, rubbers, raincoats, safes. He saw in simulated action the first condom of its kind in the United States with two unique features: (a) it had a medical-grade adhesive around its base to guard against leakage and slippage; and (b) it came with a second, temporary outer sheath over the condom itself to guard against accidental puncture by jewelry or fingernails and to make it easier to roll on in an instant.[2] "It was weird," he recalls in an interview. "With all the mechanical penises going up and down, up and down, I felt out of place being there."

Thornton, today a cheerful father of a (planned) four-year-old, thinks back to his visit to the Minneapolis condom maker as more than just another story about new technology. He found out that day that of the 3 million or so condoms purchased daily in the United States, between 40 and 70 percent are bought by females. He also found that prior to Mentor's new condom, women typically were ignored by condom makers when it came to advertising. Apparently the low-tech rubbers of the past relied on low-tech marketing research. By marrying new condom safety features with the realization that women buy millions of condoms each week, Mentor helped give old-fashioned sheaths new life. It made condoms—the new standard accessory in the 1980s and 1990s dating scene—both sexier and easier for beginners to use.

The key is in the adhesive that keeps the condom on. It makes the condom trickier to produce, but also more effective than the old condom standard of 85 to 97 percent pregnancy-proof. "We discovered that other condoms would slip off with about an ounce of pressure," a Mentor official said. "With our condom it took 280 ounces of pressure. We also discovered that at about 75 ounces of pressure the man starts screaming." The trick is to read the instructions and *roll* this new kind of condom off the penis without exerting many ounces of pressure. As in: Do Not Yank.

"I really like them," says Amy H., twenty-four, a law student from Berkeley, California. "I don't like the after-sex drip [of sperm from the vagina], so I like using condoms. But you can't trust them 100 percent. [Also,] it's so much more 'sanitary' than the pill when you consider STDs. But if I'm involved with someone, I would never say, 'You have to use a condom because I don't like that dripping feeling.' "

While women don't seem to enjoy the inconvenience of using condoms any more than men do, they sometimes get more pleasure from intercourse when condoms are used. One reason is that the decreased friction a man feels directly on the skin and nerves of his penis may result in him lasting longer before ejaculation. This might work to a couple's advantage if extended lovemaking is what they're after. Secondly women who lack vaginal lubrication during foreplay or intercourse may benefit from lubricated condoms—without having to insert K-Y jelly or other moisture-enhancing products by hand.

"It doesn't make a difference to me at all," adds Amy H., when asked how intercourse feels with a condom. "Guys will tell you, 'Oh, I can't feel anything.' But I think a lot of it's hype. A male friend told me that some of the women he's been with just *love* the feeling of a man coming inside of them, no condom, no nothing. I said, 'Yeah, right, get real.'" Yet it's true: Some women do.

BIRTH CONTROL BOX SCORE: THE CONDOM

PREGNANCY PREVENTION: 88 to 98 percent effective.
STD PREVENTION: Highly effective.
COST: Usually less than $1 per condom.
PRESCRIPTION NEEDED: No.

THE DIAPHRAGM

Of all the barrier methods of contraception, the diaphragm seems at first glance to be the most like an actual barrier. It is rubber, round, pliable, and has a sheathed wire rim for support that is sometimes spring-loaded for precise fitting. It comes in a hard plastic shell of a case that looks a lot like a clamshell. It's tough, durable. But not too tough for a woman or her partner to insert in a hurry.

When inserted correctly, a diaphragm works to prevent pregnancy in two ways. First, it covers a woman's cervix to keep sperm out. Second, its shallow, cuplike, pliable surface holds spermicide (applied prior to insertion and placed against the cervix), which creates a powerful chemical barrier as well. Some clinicians in fact tell women that the diaphragm's primary role is to keep the spermicide up against the cervix. The diaphragm is

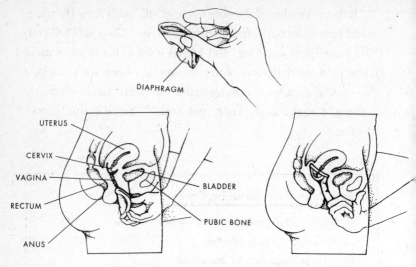

INSERTION OF A DIAPHRAGM

held securely in place along the back wall of the vagina, behind the pubic bone. For convenience, it can be inserted up to six hours before intercourse. And while it should remain in place, though, for at least six hours after having sex (to allow the spermicide to kill remaining sperm), it should not be left in for more than twenty-four hours at a time (to prevent infections from occurring).

Gynecologists typically can fit a diaphragm for a woman's vagina in five or ten minutes. What most men and a lot of women don't know about diaphragms is that they need to be refitted every once in a while, such as after a woman gives birth. In addition, sometimes after a woman's weight changes, or if she finds the muscular support around her vagina changing, she will also need to use a new size. Some women aren't able to use a diaphragm at all—if their vaginal walls can't keep the diaphragm in place or if they are uncomfortable with the process of inserting it deeply into the vagina. On rare occasions a woman may be

fitted with a larger diaphragm when a partner complains of repeatedly bumping his penis against the diaphragm rim during
intercourse.

"But even that doesn't hurt," says Anne R., thirty-two, a single
woman from Fort Lauderdale. "What does hurt is when you
leave it in like they tell you to and you end up getting a urinary
tract infection." This is a complaint often associated with diaphragm use, although gynecologists say diaphragms themselves
don't *cause* such infections. Rather, certain women are more
prone to infections if they have intercourse with different partners or sometimes even the same partner, depending on their
menstrual cycle. (It also depends on how closely she follows
directions for using and removing the diaphragm after the alotted
time.)

According to both gynecologists and diaphragm manufacturers, neither partner should notice the diaphragm during intercourse if it has been properly fitted and inserted. Women
generally use a diaphragm for about a year, at which time they
should check with their doctor about replacing it. Especially if
they have had a pelvic infection, an abortion, or weight gain or
loss of ten pounds or more. Any of these events can alter the
cervix and thus the fit of the diaphragm.

BIRTH CONTROL BOX SCORE: THE DIAPHRAGM

PREGNANCY PREVENTION: 98 percent effective (if used with
    spermicide).
STD PREVENTION: Low to none; should not be used by those who
    have had history of STDs.
COST: $100 to $150, including doctor visit for fitting. (Can be
    used for up to a year.)
PRESCRIPTION NEEDED: Yes.

THE CERVICAL CAP

The cervical cap looks like the diaphragm's little sister. Instead of heel-sized it's closer to big-toe-sized and in sex-education books is often described as thimblelike. It's both old and new, in that it was first developed in the nineteenth century, but was recently modified and approved for use in the United States in 1988. In practice a cervical cap fits tightly around a woman's cervical opening, enclosing it with suction, and forming a barrier between the vaginal canal and the uterus. To prepare a cervical cap for use, a woman slathers spermicide on the side that covers the cervix, much the way she would a diaphragm. Because it's a smaller instrument, it needs to be fitted more precisely than a diaphragm.

The main advantage of using a cervical cap as opposed to a diaphragm is that it can be inserted up to forty-eight hours before intercourse. Its effectiveness is about equal to that of a diaphragm, depending on how well it is used.[3] Since it is smaller and fits more deeply inside a woman, it is also less likely to be bumped by a thrusting penis.

A disadvantage is that it is more difficult to insert, with its small size and its use of suction to remain in place. It also can be quite tricky to remove. In addition, scattered reports of abnormal Pap smears (of cultured cervical cells) have surfaced among longtime cervical-cap users, but researchers aren't yet sure there's a connection. The abnormal Pap smears may have resulted from spermicide being held against the cervix longer than with the diaphragm. Then, too, other factors (including sexual behavior unrelated to the cervical cap) may be responsible.

In general, gynecologists in the United States don't consider the cervical cap as simple to fit or prescribe as a diaphragm. Because it is more time-consuming for them to test-fit, insert, and explain thoroughly, it is not nearly prescribed as often as other barrier methods. It's a new device here, unfamiliar to a lot of health practitioners.

Cervical caps are quite popular in Europe, though, and the reproductive-education groups Planned Parenthood and the Alan Guttmacher Institute in New York say we may start to see a large influx of cervical caps in the United States as early as 1995. Approved for use by the FDA in May 1988, cervical caps were the preferred choice of birth control for some seventy thousand women in the United States by the end of 1989.[4]

BIRTH CONTROL BOX SCORE: THE CERVICAL CAP

PREGNANCY PREVENTION: 88 to 97 percent effective (if used with spermicide).

STD PREVENTION: Moderately effective, especially for upper genital tract.

COST: $100 to $150, including doctor visit for fitting and exam.

PRESCRIPTION NEEDED: Yes.

THE CONTRACEPTIVE SPONGE

While the use of sea sponges for contraception dates back to early Egyptian times, the modern version made of synthetic materials wasn't approved for sale in the United States until 1983. Since then its popularity has increased steadily among women looking for a nonhormonal barrier method of contraception (somewhat similar to a diaphragm) that doesn't require a doctor's prescription or fitting. That "advantage"—the spontaneity and ease of use without a prescription—is also a disadvantage, however. For in terms of effectiveness in preventing pregnancy, the contraceptive sponge consistently ranks decidedly lower in preventing pregnancy than the diaphragm or cervical cap.

Using the sponge "consistently and according to label instructions," Whitehall Laboratories says, women can expect an effectiveness rate of 89 to 91 percent. But in clinical trials that (realistically) included women *who did not* use the sponge consistently and properly, the effectiveness rate ranged from 72 to 95 percent. Viewed another way, this translates to a "failure rate" as high as 28 percent. Understandably this rate may not be effective enough for a lot of couples who wish to use only one type of birth control at a time. (The maker of the Today sponge lists a toll-free telephone number on the package for users and potential customers to call for more information about the device.)

"I used the sponge only a few times and I didn't like it," says Sheri T., twenty-six and single in New York City. "I thought it was difficult and annoying. It wasn't uncomfortable, but it's messy. I didn't have any trouble positioning it, but it was pretty difficult to remove. So there you are, after having sex, sitting in the bathroom trying to get the thing out. Who wants to do that? . . . I've been on the pill for the past three months."

"It's better than the diaphragm," counters Anne R., thirty-two, of Fort Lauderdale. "I seem to get urinary tract infections with the diaphragm but not with the sponge. But I also use condoms."

The manufacturers of Today report the sponge has no or extremely low risk of infection so long as it is removed within twenty-four hours of insertion. But will sponges soon proliferate throughout the U.S. birth control market? That's not likely. While the no-mess, easy-to-use features might make this a popular method for those seeking spontaneous contraception, for established couples the sponge will more likely be used as a backup method in the future along with some other form of contraception.

BIRTH CONTROL BOX SCORE: THE SPONGE

PREGNANCY PREVENTION: 72 to 95 percent effective.

STD PREVENTION: Moderately effective, contains spermicide.

COST: $5 to $10.

PRESCRIPTION NEEDED: No.

THE IUD

The intrauterine device, or IUD, is a small piece of (usually) T-shaped plastic that is inserted by a doctor into the uterus and left in place for months at a time, up to a year. IUDs, dispensed by prescription only, may contain small amounts of copper or hormones, depending on the brand, which are released slowly over time. They usually have a long, thin filament tail. Unlike the pill, once an IUD is in place, it is immediately effective.

An IUD appears to prevent pregnancy by making the uterus an inhospitable (some doctors say "hostile") place for a fertilized egg to attach itself. But we aren't exactly sure how it works. The body of the IUD remains wholly inside the womb, while its tail runs through the cervix out of the womb into the vagina. Women use the tail to touch and check that the IUD is in place; if the string disappears, the wearer should see her doctor as soon as possible to make sure the IUD hasn't either become lodged in one of her organs or expelled.

If people today don't seem to know a lot about IUDs, chances are they have at least heard of their potential dangers. In the 1970s, when IUDs were much more popular, one brand, the Dalkon Shield, was implanted in millions of women and was later implicated in thousands of cases of painful pelvic distress, miscarriage, and fertility problems and sterility. A class-action suit resulted in years of dispute and millions of dollars in awarded claims and payments to women who had used the Dalkon Shield and suffered from it.

With this in mind, it's not surprising that some women and manufacturers remain reluctant to use or make IUDs today. Even so, it is a medical fact that IUDs have been improved markedly, and the currently available brands have passed rigorous federal testing that wasn't applied to the early 1970s versions. In addition, IUDs continue to be popular elsewhere around the world, especially in Europe, with effectiveness rates as high as 96 to 98 percent.

"These days I'm trying to procreate, procreate, procreate," says Belinda K., thirty-one, an ex-nurse with two children who now works as a medical researcher in San Diego, "but my last form of birth control was an IUD. I had it for two years and really loved it. I didn't have any problems at all. I was scared a bit by the past history, and for that reason I asked my doctor to give me low-grade antibiotics [prophylactically] to combat any possibility of infection. I got the IUD because I wanted something fail-proof. It is pretty painful to have inserted, but the pain is very short-lasting."

In regard to safety and the recurrent concern about possible pelvic infection associated with the devices, the American Medical Association scientists recently gave two currently available IUDs clean bills of health. Writing in *The Journal of the American Medical Association* in April 1989, researchers said that the Progestasert and Copper T 380 IUDs, "when used in women in monogamous relationships . . . are reliable in reducing pregnancy and have relatively few complications."[5]

However, members of the AMA panel cautioned that use of IUDs was not recommended for women who have multiple sexual partners, histories of pelvic infections, bleeding disorders, or have had ectopic pregnancies (when a fertilized egg attaches to part of a fallopian tube instead of the uterus). For women who have already had a child, are over twenty-five, and are not prone to pelvic infections, though, the IUD can be a safe and reliable means of birth control.[6]

BIRTH CONTROL BOX SCORE: IUD

PREGNANCY PREVENTION: 96 to 99 percent effective.

STD PREVENTION: Ineffective; increases the risk that any infection will spread to the uterus.

COST: $300, including doctor visit for fitting and exam.

PRESCRIPTION NEEDED: Yes.

SPERMICIDAL JELLY, CREAM, AND FOAM

Spermicidal jellies, cream, foam, and gel, despite their disparate makeup and delivery systems, share two common goals: (a) to block the opening of the cervix from advancing sperm; and (b) to kill sperm inside the vagina and render it useless. They also share a liability: If used alone, without a diaphragm, cervical cap, or condom, their effectiveness rate is about 80 to 85 percent. When used in tandem with another barrier method, though, the effectiveness of the combined contraceptives rises to, on average, 85 to 96 or 97 percent.

When using contraceptive cream or jelly without a diaphragm or cervical cap, it should be put into place (often with a plunger-type applicator that resembles a tampon in shape) before any penis-vaginal contact but as close as possible to the time of intercourse. Though thirty minutes before intercourse is all right, spermicides begin to lose their effectiveness if injected an hour or more before intercourse. The important point to remember in using all spermicides is that *they must cover the cervix to be effective;* they must be inserted as deeply as possible in the vagina. If they are inserted only into the outer part of the vagina, sperm may easily whoosh right by and reach the cervix.

While manufacturers claim their spermicides are odorless and tasteless, countless men and women who use spermicides and perform oral sex regularly report quite the opposite. Often sex educators will advise sex partners to wait until after cunnilingus, if they engage in it, to apply the spermicide. Other lovers say they don't much mind the slightly briny, metallic taste.

"It may not be the most effective method," says Anne R., thirty-two, "but I think it's the most playful. I wouldn't describe it as *fun*, but somehow it seems less serious than sticking a diaphragm in you. I've let boyfriends help me."

In fact some sex education or health books encourage a man to help his female partner with insertion of spermicides, just as a man may encourage a woman to help him roll on a condom. The former, however, may not be wise. Because even the most sensitive of male sex partners cannot *feel* the cervical opening in the same way that a woman can. No matter how diligent, he may not be able to put the jelly, foam, gel, or cream properly into place. A woman who knows her body quite well, and who has put hundreds of tampons in place, will have a better feel for how far in an applicator or plunger should be inserted in order to blanket the cervix thoroughly with spermicide.[7] That's why some family planning experts advise men to let their partners handle this particular procedure.

NATURAL OR FERTILITY AWARENESS (RHYTHM) METHODS

To many people natural birth control seems pretty unnatural. The basic idea is to predict exactly when a woman is fertile each month by *closely* monitoring her menstrual cycle. Over a period of a few months a woman (or couple) will observe the amount and kind of her slight vaginal discharge on different days, note changes in the position of her cervix, and keep track of very slight changes in body temperature during ovulation. Charts, notes on menstruation, and special thermometers all come into play.

By using natural birth control, a woman can learn to predict when she is about to ovulate. She uses this knowledge to block out certain days when unprotected intercourse is "danger-ous"—when it has a high likelihood of resulting in pregnancy. The keys to these methods, which may be only 60 to 70 percent effective if they are the sole methods used, are noting the changes in cervical mucus and body temperature—her natural rhythm.

"Either I've been lucky or I'm in touch with my cycle and not very fertile," says Laura M., thirty-eight, a single antiques dealer from Connecticut. "I've used condoms or the rhythm method for fifteen years and I've never gotten pregnant."

Using tissues or her fingers, a woman observes from time to time how the cervical mucus changes during a cycle from normally cloudy and tacky to clear and slippery when an egg is released (at ovulation). The first indication of the presence of this slick mucus, which has migrated from the cervix to the vaginal opening, is the sign to abstain from intercourse. It makes sense when you think about it: slippery mucus means sperm can more easily slip by. It follows, then, that abstinence should continue until four days after the last day the slick mucus has appeared.

In the so-called basal body temperature method, a woman takes her temperature with a special (inexpensive) thermometer each morning, then records the readings over time on a chart. (Drugstores sell basal body thermometers; gynecologists and family-planning clinics carry detailed temperature charts.) Over time the readings will show that a woman's temperature rises slightly following ovulation and remains higher until menstruation, when it begins to fall. After three days of the slightly higher temperature (as little as one-tenth of a degree Fahrenheit) the "unsafe time" is over, according to this method. On average most women will find that their fertile periods run from days 8 to 18 of their menstrual cycle.

Often used by Catholic and other women whose religious codes forbid the use of contraceptives, fertility awareness methods are also used informally by couples who want to have intercourse now and then without birth control. Or if they normally use combination methods, perhaps they will use only one during a woman's "unfertile" time. And of course fertility awareness is crucial, as Chapter 10 shows, when a couple thinks the time is right not for contraception but procreation.

BIRTH CONTROL BOX SCORE: RHYTHM METHODS
_____

PREGNANCY PREVENTION: 77 to 90 percent effective.

STD PREVENTION: Ineffective.

COST: Free (or about $10 for thermometer)

PRESCRIPTION NEEDED: No.

THE IMPLANT

Imagine six tiny time-release capsules, about the size of matches, that are implanted in a fanlike pattern in a woman's upper arm by her biceps and you have an idea of what one of the newest contraceptives in America is all about. The Norplant, as it's called, was approved by the FDA for use in the United States in late 1990. This contraceptive requires minor surgery to make the implant, which remains in place and is effective for up to five years, or until a woman wants it removed. Over time the implant slowly releases synthetic progestin that is similar to what is contained in the birth control pills that contain progestin but no estrogen.

According to gynecologists who've studied its use in Europe and other countries (where it's been available for years), the implant should meet the contraception needs of millions of women who seek effective long-term birth control but who shouldn't take the pill or who aren't ready for sterilization. The implant is almost instantly reversible if a woman changes her mind about wanting children, yet this again requires minor surgery.

Because the implant doesn't contain estrogen, it may pose less long-term risk of cardiovascular problems to users than some types of the pill. Although users have reported menstrual irregularities after having the implant, a woman's cycle usually returns to normal after a few months.

At a spring 1990 public briefing on new forms of birth control, Dr. George Thomas of Mount Sinai Medical Center in New York City said those who would be well suited for the implant include women who want long-term birth spacing, women who have had physical problems with other contraceptives, women who need to avoid estrogen, and in some cases women who have repeatedly used abortion as birth control. Those who shouldn't use the implant include women who report irregular bleeding, women who have had breast cancer or liver problems; and women who suspect they may be pregnant.

In terms of effectiveness, Thomas says reputable studies have shown that the implant has prevented pregnancy 98.4 to 99.8 percent of the time. These extremely high efficiency rates coupled with the no-worry, almost-no-maintenance features, suggest that these tiny capsules will be quite popular as contraceptives in the United States before long. Even with the prospect of minor surgery and a price tag (including the implant procedure) of $500, the implant will be deemed well worth its cost if it lives up to the lofty reputation that's preceded it so far.

BIRTH CONTROL BOX SCORE: THE IMPLANT

PREGNANCY PREVENTION: 98 to 99 percent effective.

STD PREVENTION: Low; doesn't protect against gonorrhea or chlamydia, but does thicken cervical mucus, which protects upper genital tract against pelvic inflammatory disease.

COST: About $500 for implants that last for five years, office visit, and surgical procedure.

PRESCRIPTION NEEDED: Yes.

STERILIZATION

It comes as a surprise to many people that sterilization is the most popular form of birth control among *married* people in the United States. A 1988 National Center for Health Statistics study showed a sterilization rate among females aged fifteen to forty-four of 16.6 percent, compared with about 13 percent of women of that age in 1982. It is also almost always irreversible surgery, with an effectiveness rate of preventing pregnancy of over 99 percent (in a very few cases the operation isn't totally successful).

When a woman opts for sterilization, one or two incisions are made in her lower abdomen, depending on the type of procedure, and her fallopian tubes are surgically cut or blocked. This prevents an egg from ever again meeting or being fertilized by sperm. This is known as tubal ligation. The three most common types of ligation sterilization for women are: (1) laparoscopy; (2) minilaparotomy ("minilap"); and (3) vaginal sterilization. Each one differs markedly from the simpler, less-risky, and less-invasive vasectomy procedure for men. In a vasectomy the thin sperm-carrying tubes, the vas deferens, are snipped and tied back. These two tubes, which lead from the testicles to the urethra, are carefully pulled out of the scrotum through half-inch incisions and then cut, in an office procedure or clinical setting, using local anesthesia. This prevents sperm from ever again mixing with a man's seminal fluid, though he will still ejaculate in other ways as before. Approximately 7 percent of American men now choose to be sterilized, and the number has recently been rising.

Although women sometimes opt for local or spinal anesthesia during sterilization, most tubal ligation is done under general anesthesia. In addition, female sterilization almost always involves more complicated surgery than that of a vasectomy. That said, women who get sterilized or "have their tubes tied" will find that their ovaries and uterus don't change; their eggs can simply no longer be fertilized by sperm.

(1) A laparoscopy is so named for an instrument, the laparoscope, which is inserted through an incision beneath the navel and which contains a fiber-optic camera device for precise viewing of the fallopian tubes. With the pelvic organs in sight, the doctor makes another incision just above the pubic-hair line and inserts the other instrument, a cutting or clamping tool, used to seal off the tubes. The operation is usually done in thirty minutes, barring complications.

(2) A minilaparotomy is the simplest female sterilization procedure (in theory), because it involves making only one incision, one to three inches long above the pubic-hair line, through which the doctor manually removes the tubes, closes them off, and then sutures the incision. Again, the procedure usually is done in thirty minutes, barring complications.

(3) Vaginal sterilization is tricky to perform, even for experienced physicians, because there is no incision made in the abdomen or above the pubic bone. It's done through the vagina. But women who opt for vaginal sterilization do so largely because there are no visible scars. Instead, after a speculum is put in place to hold the vagina open, a doctor makes an incision in the back wall of the vagina, through which he or she then inserts an instrument to reach and close off the fallopian tubes. This type of tubal ligation can be done in thirty minutes or less and is most likely to be successful if a woman's uterus, tubes, and ovaries are relatively mobile (and free of infection and prior scarring) and if her pelvic muscles are fairly lax. Vaginal sterilization also carries a slightly higher risk of infection than other procedures because of the bacteria normally present in the vagina itself.

After laparoscopy or minilaparotomy most women can return home within six hours of the procedure. Those having vaginal sterilizations usually remain in a hospital overnight for observation, as do others who have had more complicated sterilization surgeries than the three mentioned above.

BIRTH CONTROL BOX SCORE: STERILIZATION

PREGNANCY PREVENTION: 99.7 percent effective.

STD PREVENTION: None.

COST: $300 to $500 including doctor visit.

PRESCRIPTION NEEDED: Not applicable.

ABORTION

It is of course a controversial method of controlling birth and it isn't at all simple. But the fact remains, as many as 1.5 million women and teenagers undergo legal abortions each year in the United States. Once an unwanted pregnancy has been confirmed by a doctor, a woman who chooses to have an abortion should move swiftly. The sooner the abortion is done, the lower the risk of medical complications associated with it.

As might be expected, abortions performed in the first trimester are the safest of all. Medically speaking, the first trimester refers to the first thirteen weeks of pregnancy, dating back to the first day of the last menstrual period. The second trimester refers to the fourteenth through the twenty-fourth weeks; the third trimester is twenty-five weeks and more into the pregnancy.

For those unfamiliar with abortion procedures, it might help to think of abortion in three stages: (1) preparation of the vagina, cervix, and uterus (including anesthesia and disinfectant); (2) removal of the embryo or fetus and lining of the uterus; and (3) removal of instruments and beginning of recovery.

There are a number of different abortion procedures, but the method most often performed by far is vacuum aspiration, or early vacuum abortion. This involves inserting a speculum to keep the vagina open, a clamp (tenaculum) to keep the cervix (leading to the uterus) steady, and a series of dilating instruments to open the cervix gradually. When the cervix is dilated to a sufficient diameter, the doctor inserts a thin vacuum tube into the uterus and vacuums out the pregnancy sac and its contents. Then he or she inspects the uterus to make certain the tissues have been removed. Even in early-trimester abortions, women report feeling tugging sensations in their abdomens and painful cramping after the procedure is done.

"I was nineteen when I had my abortion, and I was ten weeks pregnant," says Anne R., of Fort Lauderdale. "It was during college. My boyfriend drove me to the clinic, then dropped me off. It felt cold, mechanical, scary, and I was in a fog during the whole thing. It definitely hurt, even though I was drugged up. I can't say it was traumatic in a specific sense, but I was sick, bloated, pregnant, and, like I said, I was in pain."

Abortions performed after thirteen weeks of pregnancy involve more preparation, slightly greater risk of complications, and larger instruments entering the uterus through the cervix. The most frequently performed procedures in the second trimester are dilation and curettage (D & C), dilation and evacuation (D & E), and induction abortion.

A D & C involves dilating the cervical opening, then scraping out the uterine lining, including the pregnancy (fetal) tissues. (D & Cs are also performed in normal gynecological procedures for treating various uterine problems unrelated to pregnancy.) A D & E is a newer abortion method that is part D & C and part vacuum aspiration. It is more complicated than a simple D & C, but it also is more effective and may be less painful. Induction abortion involves injecting a drug or drugs through the abdomen into the amniotic sac surrounding the fetus, which results in contractions and expulsion. This is followed by a D & C and typically requires a one- to two-day hospital stay.

Beyond the physical pain a woman endures from abortion, there are frequently powerful aftereffects of the procedure. In 1990, on assignment for *Esquire* magazine, author Mark Baker asked men ranging in age from twenty-eight to forty-six about how they felt after their girlfriends or wives had an abortion:

> "[Y]ou see your wife's body changing," one man said. "It changes so fast [once she's pregnant]. Her breasts get larger immediately. Her nipples get brown. . . . So it's not invisible. That's why abortion's so difficult. If there weren't physical evidence that something was going on, it might be easier to handle. You might be able to keep it in the realm of fantasy."[8]

When I asked Mike D., a twenty-eight-year-old married man from the Detroit area, what he remembered about the abortions he went through with a girlfriend in the 1980s, he said, "When you get there, you understand why some guys can't handle it. You're in the waiting room for a couple hours and you just feel stupid. Especially me, who went through it twice. I was worried about what it might do to Kim's body, so I got into a discussion with this doctor. He told me not to worry, that in Europe a lot of people use abortion as birth control; they have them over and over. I felt worse after he said that.

"I felt like I shared her pain," Mike added. "I shared the responsibility for causing her the pain." Mike also said sex with Kim after the second abortion was never quite the same. "It's not that it felt evil," he said, "but I felt like I did damage there, and here I am coming back for more."

However you look at the procedure, the more you know about abortion and its aftermath, the greater the chance that—should the need ever arise—you'll have to help your partner thoughtfully through a medical event that is, in the end, something more.

RU-486

It may be called the abortion pill, but the drug RU-486 is both simpler than an abortion procedure and at the same time more complex. First, it is actually *three* pills, which work together to end a pregnancy. In France, where it originated and where it is most widely used, RU-486 is also followed up with a prostaglandin hormone, which is taken two days after the first pills are swallowed. This hormone is used to induce contractions of the uterus. In turn these contractions will eventually lead a woman to expel, 96 percent of the time, a four- to seven-week-old embryo. While more than 45,000 women took RU-486 in the first two years after its introduction in France in 1988, the procedure is not as matter-of-fact as many people in the United States believe. The government requires that women meet with psychologists before they can take the drug, and a seven-day waiting period before taking it is also enforced.

But it works. And it is not nearly as invasive as a dilation and curettage (D & C) abortion or a suction-type abortion. Women who have used it to date have reported that they have felt more in control of their bodies and their minds than they did when they had previous abortions. Others have been surprised by the persistent pain that lingered for days.

How does it work? In brief, RU-486 discourages a fertilized egg from attaching itself to the walls of the uterus. The drug also encourages the uterus itself to slough away the egg, as it does in a menstrual period, except that this "sloughing" is chemically induced.

The downside of taking a series of pills in order to end a pregnancy has both physiological and psychological components. The physiological ones include cramping (sometimes severe) and heavy bleeding well after the embryo is expelled (up to seven to ten days). Then, in the cases where RU-486 happens to fail, a full abortion would need to be performed.

By mid-1991 more than sixty thousand women in France and elsewhere had safely aborted their pregnancies with RU-486. But France's health ministry also reported that one woman died from heart failure in early 1991 related to the procedure after being injected with the follow-up hormone, a prostaglandin called Sylorostone. She was thirty-one, in her thirteenth week of pregnancy, and was a heavy smoker. Health officials have recommended against using RU-486 when a woman smokes or when she has heart problems, but they were nonetheless shocked by the thirty-one-year-old woman's death. As a result they'll be studying different follow-up drugs to use with RU-486 for years to come.

When two journalists and a photographer from *Life* followed a "typical" French woman through the entire RU-486 process to see exactly how it turned out, the thirty-six-year-old mother of three said in the June 1990 issue that she was pleased with the procedure but surprised at the emotional burden it placed on her. Fatima (her last name was not used) spent one week pondering the procedure after an initial checkup; one hour in the clinic to take the pills; two days waiting for her next visit, at which she received a shot of prostaglandin in her left buttock; then a few hours waiting to expel the fertilized egg. She then underwent a couple of days of cramping and menstrual-type bleeding for more than a week. This was considered a longer-than-usual reaction, but not out of the reported boundaries that have been recorded so far. The point is, taking RU-486 is not merely popping a couple pills and out you go.

In the end, if you put aside the moral-ethical debates about whether taking an "abortion" pill constitutes an abortion, what remains is that RU-486 (named in part for the French manufacturer, Rousell-Uecliff) blurs the line between abortion and contraception. And that line has moved outside of France, to Sweden, China, and Great Britain, even though it has not yet reached the United States other than in tests. Chances are that due to the continuing controversy sparked by RU-486, we may not see it become available in the United States before the mid-1990s.

THE BIRTH CONTROL OF TOMORROW

Looking back, in early 1990, you could say that Congresswoman Pat Schroeder of Colorado was more than a little frustrated with the snail's pace of birth control research in the United States. "A lot of women," Schroeder said, "are using the same kind of contraceptives that Cleopatra used—sponges." Schroeder was speaking before a Planned Parenthood conference on contraceptives and their future; she hoped to leave feeling less frustrated.

And yet her fellow conferees agreed that the outlook for new contraceptives in America looked partly cloudy at best. The fear of lawsuits against manufacturers and drug companies is stifling development of new birth control devices. So is the lack of government funding. Add in antiabortion pressures that filter down through family-planning group budgets (such as Planned Parenthood's), and you begin to understand why one New York City gynecologist said recently, "We may as well be a Third World country as far as contraception is concerned."

The following research projects in birth control are now playing at a laboratory near you. Look for them at your local gynecologist's office, perhaps in the next decade.

• *The Vaginal Ring:* This device, which resembles a doughnut, or a diaphragm without its middle, fits into the vagina like a diaphragm but with a difference: The ring contains low levels of hormones, which are time-released over three to four months. A woman keeps the ring inside for three weeks, then removes it during her period. It is close to being approved for use in England.

• *Male Contraceptives:* The problem with the male pills that have been developed so far is that when they have stopped fertilization (in animal tests), they have also caused impotence. The more hopeful means for men, while not expected to reach the market by the mid-1990s, is injectable hormones. These hormones would shut down sperm production, but *not* reduce the sex-drive aspects of testosterone. Tests of these injectables are being conducted on humans at an early stage by Contraceptive Research and Development (CONRAD) in Reston, Virginia.

• *One-Year Implants:* Similar to Norplant but designed for shorter terms, implants for one year's use or less already are being tested in the United States by a biomedical research group, Family Health International, in North Carolina. The big difference from other implants? These would be biodegradable in the body, like dissolving sutures.

• *Birth Control Patches:* These are similar to the drug-dispensing, Band-Aid–type patches already used for some medications. Researchers hope to be able to synthesize estrogen and progestin into a contraceptive patch that would be "worn" on the body and changed once a week. It would mimic the effects of the pill while bypassing the digestive system completely. Thus the need for surgery (as with Norplant implants) would be bypassed as well.

• *Female Condoms:* If male pills are indeed around the corner, then the "female condom" has fairly arrived. One version, a polyethylene pouch that resembles an hourglass-shaped Baggie, received a recommendation for FDA approval by the FDA's own Obstetrics and Gynecology Devices Panel in early 1992. And while debate over what these devices should be called continues, one point is beyond debate: If and when it receives widespread approval from the FDA, the female condom will be the first new product marketed to help prevent the spread of AIDS since the disease came to light in the early 1980s.

CONTRARY PERCEPTIONS OF CONTRACEPTION

Because the primary purpose of all these devices and techniques is to control birth, it is worth taking one last look at "control." As a man you've seen that you can control certain parts of the childbirth equation, but only those leading up to conception. After that your partner will, by design, become the controlling partner of the pregnancy. So if you like to think of your relationship as equal, then you might want to get more involved in the pregnancy-planning stages. If so, you might make a conscious effort to take more responsibility for monitoring the birth control phases of your lovemaking. If you do, the evidence suggests, your efforts won't likely be overlooked:

"It's almost unfair to say that guys are irresponsible about birth control," says Belinda K., thirty-one, of San Diego, "because in the long run the woman is the one to face the consequences. But ideally it would be nice if they did know more and care."

"Condoms don't help my sex life much," says Debbie M., twenty-five, of Boston. "A lot of times Steve will lose his erection just pulling out and putting one on, although he's gotten better. He's more prepared; he tries to open the plastic wrapper before we even get started. You can also have fun putting it on.

"One time he went in, and I said, 'Wait a minute! You have to put on a condom.' And he had done it already—and it was great. I didn't have to know about it. You like your birth control to be as unobtrusive as possible. That's why I like the pill," Debbie says.

"But any birth control is nice so that he doesn't have to pull out."

BIRTH CONTROL CHOICES: WHO USES WHAT?

	1988 (in percent)	1991 (in percent)
Birth control pill	24	28
Female sterilization	14	15
Male sterilization	10	10
Condom	12	16
Withdrawal	4	5
Rhythm/Natural	3	3
Diaphragm	4	3
Sponge	2	2
IUD	1	1
No Method/Other	24	19

> > > > > Based on 62 percent
response to a questionnaire sent to
12,500 women;
Source: Ortho Pharmaceuticals, 1991.

CHAPTER 10

PREGNANCY AND CHILDBIRTH

FOR MEN

The modern man is determined to share as much as he can in pregnancy and birth. He enjoys his wife changing shape and the reality of the baby kicking against his hand.

—SHEILA KITZINGER
The Complete Book of Pregnancy and Childbirth

During pregnancy, a woman's body can respond more floridly to sexual arousal; all impulses and sensations become heightened due to the high levels of circulating sex hormones.

—DR. MIRIAM STOPPARD
The Magic of Sex

While most of this book explores recreational sex and sexual health, this chapter looks at the aftereffects of *pro*creational sex—from conception through childbirth. But unlike most writing about pregnancy, this chapter views pregnancy from a male perspective.

No matter how much you may know about pregnancy, you have probably overlooked some numbers. And when you stop to look at them, pregnancy itself approaches a statistical miracle. Consider a man's contribution: In the course of adulthood, a man might have an average of one hundred orgasms per year, multiplied by, say, forty years of "prime" sexual activity. Which amounts to four thousand or so orgasms, give or take a few hundred, that he may enjoy in the prime of his sexual life.

If you multiply the number of sperm in an average ejaculation, 1 million (a conservative figure, sexologists say) by those four thousand orgasms, you arrive at a figure of approximately 4 billion spermatozoa ejaculated into vaginas, other orifices, condoms, bedsheets, thin air, or elsewhere. That's *4,000,000,000* sperm cells. (That's *conservative*.) And yet less than one in a billion, judging from average family-size data in the United States, connects with its feminine counterpart, a ripened egg, and becomes a child.

So when a man's partner becomes pregnant, when one of those potentially billions of sperm cells has latched onto an egg released by her ovaries (one of roughly *40,000* she is born with), and pierced its protective shell, you could say something rather extraordinary has occurred. On average, studies show that 25 percent of all couples trying to conceive will achieve this goal within the first month. By the end of a year between 85 and 90 percent of those trying to conceive will have succeeded.[1]

"The most amazing part of all this," says Paula K., thirty-four, of Princeton, New Jersey, and mother of an eighteen-month-old, "is that, I swear, I felt myself conceive. I went, 'Oh, my God!' It felt like a little tiny spark inside, a little tiny explosion, like a star bursting. I said to my husband, 'I just conceived!!' He went, 'Huh?' I was pregnant once before and had an abortion—but I felt the actual conception both times. It's unmistakable."

"I couldn't believe how easy it was for us," a thirty-year-old, first-time father from the Midwest told me about his and his wife's conception (she was twenty-eight). "After being married for two years we decided to stop using birth control, and maybe try to have a kid, and BOOM! Five weeks later we found out she was pregnant."

Boom! From that moment on, assuming a couple brings the baby to term (as this couple did), their lives will forever be altered. And the numbers don't let up: *40* weeks for an average pregnancy; *27* pounds as the average amount of weight gained by a new mother; *three* distinct stages of labor; *$5,000* for a normal hospital delivery; .5 liter (16.5 ounces) of blood lost during a normal delivery, *one* liter if it's a cesarean section;[2] and 7 pounds 6 ounces as the average weight of a newborn baby in the United States, according to the National Institute of Child and Human Development.

As a man prepares for fatherhood, however "easy" the conception, the hard part for his partner (despite the mind-numbing math) is just beginning. Her hormones quickly surge, pumping out estrogen and sending potent signals throughout her body. These in turn instruct her uterus to expand and tell her circulatory system to start increasing its blood supply in order to nourish the emerging embryo. A momentous nine-month countdown has begun.

To be sure, numbers only take you so far. From the start it's helpful to remember that every pregnancy is unique and does not necessarily follow anyone's schedule. A "normal" pregnancy, from the medical experts' perspective, can run from 240 to 300 days. It makes more sense, though, to think in terms of weeks of a pregnancy. Gestation periods of 34 to 43 weeks are considered normal, with the norm among births in the United States today at 40. As far as predicting a precise delivery date (which is projected forward 280 days from the first day of the expectant mother's last menstrual period), even the best doctors fare worse than rookie Las Vegas bookmakers. Fewer than 10 percent of women actually give birth on the day a practitioner figured upon at the outset.[3]

The briefing of bodily changes that follows is a loose list, a primer of sorts, and it includes more possibilities than one pregnant woman will probably face during pregnancy. Still, the more a man knows about what his pregnant partner is about to undergo, the more support he is able to offer. Up to a point. . . .

"Sure, he's supportive," expectant mothers say of their mates. "He supports the idea of *me* going through all this pain and discomfort for *our* baby." The jokes do, however, contain elements of truth. For all of men's involvement in the pregnancy process over the past two decades (when men began moving into the delivery rooms in large numbers), there simply is no male analog to a woman's experience of childbirth.

That said, expectant fathers can do what they can do. They can read up on the process, from nutrition to obstetrics; they can "keep the charts"—or organize a pregnancy-medical history file for their partners; they can attend classes in childbirth willingly.

When it came time for Robin P. and her husband, John, to attend Lamaze childbirth-education classes, Robin says her husband was cynical at first, abrasively so. "He should have paid more attention in class," she says. "He shouldn't have joked around so much. I think it may have been his way of dealing with insecurities, of not really knowing what was going on with my body. He always likes to be in charge, and maybe he felt like he couldn't do that there and then. But I was glad he kept telling me, 'Don't worry. When I need to, when the time comes, I take things real seriously. I'll *be* there.' "

What else can expectant fathers do for their partners? They can cook "for the three of us" (if it's a first-time pregnancy); or they can do all the above and head into the delivery room with as much confidence as a man could reasonably be expected to assume. Which means they've also got to be honest with their partners and admit when they're unsure of themselves, or unsure about the impending state of parenthood. At the very least, a man can truly share with his partner the emotional side of giving birth.

"He was wonderful," says Colleen H., thirty, of Atlanta, of her husband, Scott, reflecting on her pregnancy not quite a year ago.

"He waited on me hand and foot. Physically my life got rougher once I'd gained weight. But he had no problem cooking dinner for us, and actually he was a pain in the ass about it. He wanted to be so sure I ate the right things that he watched just about *every bite* I took. His heart was in the right place, though. He wouldn't even let me carry groceries."

A NEW LOOK AT INFERTILITY

Technically speaking, approximately 15 percent of all couples trying to have a baby are defined as being infertile—meaning they're unable to conceive after trying for one year.[4] Unfortunately couples who can't conceive often tend to think in terms of "blame," about which partner's parts are responsible for a failure to conceive. The first thing the couple should know is that among *all* couples conception and fertility is actually a chancy thing. In fact a couple has only a 20 percent probability of conceiving in any given month. When you then consider the advanced age at which many couples try to conceive in the United States today, the reasons for some prevalent problems become apparent. Dr. Stephen L. Corson, director of the Philadelphia Fertility Center, says that the birth rate among women age thirty-five and over has increased nearly 50 percent compared with births in that age range around 1980.

Not surprisingly, fertility wanes with age, yet many women today attempt to become first-time mothers in their thirties. As explained in Chapter 8, conditions such as endometriosis tend to increase in frequency among women who delay their first pregnancy. Sociologically speaking, this country has experienced a radical shift among couples in family planning over just the past twenty years. It is no coincidence that the Congressional Office of Technology Assessment has reported that in the late 1960s, about 500,000 women each year made office visits for fertility-related problems. In the late 1980s the number reached 1.6 million per year.

The other important fact to consider in infertility today is that doctors who treat the condition are increasingly looking at men (and their sperm) as potential sources of the problem. Fertility specialists estimate that men are responsible for some 30 to 40 percent of the cases of infertility that are treated. Only recently have doctors become aware of this significant number. Unfortunately many women undergo surgery for apparent fertility problems without having their husbands tested, according to information counselors at RESOLVE, a Massachusetts-based infertility support group.

The point is, infertility isn't any one person's fault. Once a couple is deemed infertile, there are numerous choices to make, from artificial insemination, fertility-boosting drugs, in-vitro fertilization ("harvesting" one of a woman's eggs, then fertilizing it in a petri dish and inserting it into the uterus), or manipulating sperm, the sperm count, or sperm motility (movement). Just as infertility isn't any one person's fault, neither is it one person's problem. These days both partners can contribute to the solution. A man can start by volunteering, early on, to have his sperm tested. Not only is this prudent from a medical standpoint, it may also save him and his partner a lot of money on inconclusive obstetrical exams.[5]

THE FIRST TRIMESTER (WEEKS 1 TO 12)

When infertility isn't a problem, or once it's been resolved, the first and most universal sign of pregnancy is a missed menstrual period. What men don't often know, though, is that many women do still bleed for a month or two even *after* they're pregnant. (Likewise, all missed periods do not mean a woman is pregnant.) On average these postconception episodes of bleeding tend to be briefer and have much less blood than a normal menstruation.

Another nearly universal early sign of pregnancy is swelling of the breasts, which may also become more tender. Often a woman's nipples become broader and the surrounding areola can darken in color, as the earliest stage of milk production begins. Her blood volume also begins to increase. One of the changes that is unseen and largely unfelt is the expansion of the uterus, a muscular organ that grows from its normal, fist-sized, one-eighth-of-a-pound size to about two and one-quarter pounds by the end of the pregnancy.

During the first twelve weeks of pregnancy the infamous morning sickness may strike any number of times. It could manifest as a mild queasiness or be strong enough to cause vomiting. But regardless of the conventional wisdom, not all women get morning sickness. Your wife or partner may also have to urinate more frequently because of internal hormonal changes and the added pressure placed on the bladder by the expanding womb. Constipation may also occur, caused by hormones and, later, by the constriction of the intestines due to pressure placed on them by the growth of the fetus. Headaches and extreme fatigue, too, may join the fray. All this can sound oppressive, especially to a man who's not feeling any of this himself. Of course it doesn't happen all at once. And it doesn't *all* happen to every woman with child. But it can be oppressive.

"Sometimes you get to feeling so overwhelmed by being pregnant," says Colleen H. "And even though that's in the [pregnancy] books, it's easy to gloss over. You think, 'My life is not my own—it's killin' me!' It demands all your time, every minute of the day. At least it felt that way."

Unlike a number of women I spoke with, Robin P., of Phoenix, says her husband's view of her pregnant body was incredibly warm and supportive, bordering on worshipful. "We were newly married," she says, "and before we got married, I had been working out a lot at my health club. My body was in shape, and it held up while I was pregnant. John would say, 'I think you look great!' Or, 'That's just your stomach, you look beautiful.' He concentrated a lot on my breasts, and it was weird how he seemed proud of them. He even bragged to his sister a couple times about how they had leaked milk. I reminded him it's not *that* special; it's what animals do in the wild. It's weird, though. My first husband didn't like the fact that they leaked sometimes. He couldn't deal with that, and I wanted him to have a better attitude about it."

"He was sensitive to my body but not always to my mind," says Paula K., describing how her husband reacted throughout her pregnancy. "He's older than I am, and he has two kids in their twenties that he'd had from his first marriage. But men didn't get nearly as involved in the pregnancy or delivery back then.

"You know," adds Paula, "I don't really consider my husband to have been there during my pregnancy—I never felt he was really there with me. But during delivery he was there 100 percent, maybe 200 percent. I think it's kind of a male thing. They react to a crisis, but during the first nine months they feel helpless a lot of the time."

"Fathers don't always understand how she [the mother] can feel so terrible," says Margaret Truesdale, R.N., a childbirth educator for twenty-two years who has taught hundreds of expectant parents about deliveries and Lamaze breathing techniques at Boston's Beth Israel Hospital. "They don't get why she can't take a deep breath toward the end of the pregnancy, why she has to go to the bathroom so often, and why he often eats alone."

Men can help counteract these feelings in a couple of ways: by accompanying their partner on visits to the obstetrician if possible; by making a few opportune trips to the local library in search of specific articles or books (such as *What to Expect When*

You're Expecting) that deal with their partner's problem or stage of pregnancy; or they can interview a number of their co-workers (male and female), friends, and family members about their pregnancies, past and present. These are small steps, perhaps, but they are things a man can do to soften some of the pain, to face down some of the fears.

"I think *men* need to be cared for a lot during pregnancy," says Rosemary Diliu, director of parent-education programs at the Maternity Center Association, a New York–based, not-for-profit health care agency founded back in 1918. "In fact, when they come in with their wives or partners for the exams, we sometimes take their blood pressure too. A man doesn't want to be left out of this event," Diliu says. "He wants to be more than a sperm donor."

"My husband, Don, got incredibly involved the first time I got pregnant," says Tina D., twenty-eight, a mother of three who lives in a Chicago suburb. "I mean he would *read* those baby books." She laughs. "He was so incredibly *boring:* 'It's a month-and-a-half now,' he'd say, 'and the baby is now the size of a grain of rice. . . .' I don't think he's a normal guy in the way he gets into this stuff." Tina likes poking fun at her husband, but it's obvious in her voice she's glad he *is* "into this stuff."

BY WEEK 8

Although by the fourth week of pregnancy there are hardly any outward signs that a woman is in fact pregnant, weeks 4 through 8 are remarkable in their *internal* efficiency. For by week 8, all of the baby's inner organs are present. They are not perfectly formed or developed, but they're there. At the same time, the bones begin to develop, which makes sense when you consider that one of the lifelong functions of human bone is to protect the internal organs.

Another widely reported physiological change during early

pregnancy is that secretions of the vagina may seem and feel different (to both partners). This occurs because the chemical makeup of the vagina changes markedly. In addition to extra estrogen, progesterone is also released during pregnancy, as is the pregnancy hormone, HCG, or human chorionic gonadotropin. In light of all this activity, a woman may become more susceptible to yeast infections during this time.

Mark N., thirty-two, a father-to-be from the Baltimore area, can attest to this unabashedly. He recently spoke about what he'd learned about having oral sex with his sixteen-weeks-pregnant wife. "We do it, but it's not so great right now." Some men (and women) find these vaginal changes sexy, and literally life-enhancing. Others are turned off by unfamiliar sights and smells in such an intimate area. As we'll see later in this chapter, sex during pregnancy, for a number of reasons, takes on a life of its own.

"Everything's so different now," Mark said. "My little penis and my little tongue can't do much down there. It's as if [the vagina] is saying, 'Get out of here. We're busy now.' And my wife even told me, 'You probably don't want to go down there.' "

THE SECOND TRIMESTER (WEEKS 13 TO 26)

In contrast to the first, the second trimester of a woman's pregnancy is normally more pleasant and forgiving. Her hormone surges will have settled some, and the burdensome fatigue of the first twelve weeks usually dissipates during these middle weeks.

Likewise, breast tenderness tends to diminish, as do most of the nagging pangs associated with morning sickness. By about the sixteenth week of pregnancy the uterus has enlarged to the size of a large grapefruit. By now a woman may feel the first sensations of what seems like butterflies in her stomach. These are, in fact, the first signs of movement by the fetus.

Some women say they feel a kind of glow of well-being during the second trimester. It is probably a reaction to their adjustment to the new levels of estrogen, progesterone, and pregnancy hormone that have been zinging about in their bodies. Yet even as some say they feel a "glow" on the inside, they scowl at their outside as their waist begins to bloat. To many pregnant women negative thoughts about body image (see Chapter 3) may rise anew, adding emotional pressure to a time when added girth and weight gain *should* be signs of life and celebration.

"I got backrubs from my husband," Paula K. says, "but I practically had to beg for them. And they felt great because everything hurts all the time. You can't get comfortable and you're waddling around. You can't sleep, you can't see your feet. I do think that it would have helped if he'd given me more physical empathy."

A male partner facing this unease may find the most helpful reaction is to be honest—to acknowledge the extra weight his partner is carrying and to thank her for the physical work she is doing for them and their baby. He can also begin to take more responsibility for initiating massages or sex play that may have been infrequent or absent during the first trimester. Many women find warm (but not too hot, for reasons of fetal safety) baths relaxing during these weeks, especially if their partner joins them in the tub or attends to them with a soapy sponge.

BY WEEK 20

Moving through her second trimester, an expectant mother may sweat more, and her skin may develop ruddy stretch marks and become drier. The area around her nipples tends to darken, as does the region of her lower abdomen. By week 20 or 22 a woman's breasts are nearly ready for nursing her newborn. At this point a yellowish fluid known as colostrum may at times be secreted by the nipples; it is not a cause for alarm but merely a precursor to breast milk and breast-feeding.

With the extra weight a woman is carrying, she may develop spidery varicose veins on her legs or midsection. These are actually nothing more than dilated blood vessels, and for the most part they will recede after delivery, but probably not completely. Similarly most pregnant women develop hemorrhoids, a kind of varicose vein and swelling in and around the anus, another result of added weight and pressure on an area of the body not usually stressed in this manner. These, too, will subside, usually within a couple of months of delivery.

The fetus reaches the so-called quickening stage by week 20, which prompts the mother's first definite "I felt it *move*." (The first faint fluttering movements are felt between weeks 15 and 18.) The fetus has made it through the most tenuous time, the first trimester. The risks of miscarriage and severe injury to the fetus begin to taper off starting at about week 13. Later, toward the end of the second trimester, the fetal brain begins its most significant period of growth. A little life is being primed.

THE THIRD TRIMESTER

Weeks 27 through 40 are at once precarious and thrilling—for this is when a baby undergoes its final biological primping before its birth. By week 28, measuring about 14 inches and weighing approximately 2 pounds, the baby is considered viable, meaning that if delivered at this stage, it is required to be registered by hospital authorities.[6]

The major organ systems were formed in the first two trimesters; now is the time when they mature to enable the infant to survive outside the womb. During this trimester a woman may sometimes feel as if she's lost control of her body. It is still enlarging, pressing out, and everything inside feels even tighter now, again causing a host of discomforts that don't seem to subside. For instance, shortness of breath may occur even *in the absence* of exercise or mildly strenuous effort.

BY WEEK 35

By week 35 a woman may feel as if she's a prisoner of her body, even as she sleeps. Due to lower back pain she may not be able to sleep on her back—and in fact many doctors caution women not to. This is because the uterus may put pressure on the main abdominal blood vessels, which deliver the baby's supply of blood and nourishment. Sleeping on her side, then, with pillows propped up and against her, may be the best and most comfortable alternative. Obstetricians often encourage women to take naps during the day to make up for lost sleep at night ("You're not just eating for two, you're sleeping for two as well").

As for her overall body shape a fullness may set in that is both physically and emotionally distorting. Known as edema, this swelling occurs most often in the legs, especially around the ankles and the feet. And because this can get quite uncomfortable for women who must stand a lot (during work or at other times), doctors encourage them to take breaks, keep moving, and keep the blood coursing through both their own body and the umbilical cord to the fetus.

Prior to childbirth the uterus, which feels hard to the touch now, almost like a shell, will tighten sporadically and without apparent provocation. These episodes, known as Braxton-Hicks contractions, are often frightening to pregnant women and their husbands at first because they mimic the first pangs of labor. They are a harmless, natural occurrence, though, and are thought to help strengthen and prepare the uterus for imminent delivery.

"We were four weeks early, and we thought labor had started," one twenty-eight-year-old father from Missouri told me, recounting the weeks before the birth of his baby son, "so we raced to the hospital at four A.M. They told us these were Braxton-Hicks contractions—which hadn't been as strong before. It was false labor, but I was glad we went to the hospital anyway; I was freaking out . . . it was so early."

Emotionally the last few weeks of pregnancy can be taxing in their own right. A woman may complain about feeling as if she'll be pregnant forever, and yet she may also prefer this "annoyed" state to what actually lies ahead—the unknown (and perhaps frightening) phases of labor and childbirth. It's a dilemma for both male and female partners, for the man may say he under-stands while he doesn't really. The best he can do is to *try* to understand these mixed emotions in the context of months of her physical discomfort. He can also take over the more mundane household chores from this point until delivery, to ease the body and mind of his partner. It's a start.

CHILDBIRTH REVISITED

"I just don't think men have any idea how much pain a woman goes through during childbirth," says Marcus H., twenty-seven, a father of a five-month-old from Washington, D.C., thinking back to the day of his son's birth. "You can go to the Lamaze classes, read all the books, talk to other women who've had babies, but it's just not the same as being there while she's going through it. It was unbelievable.

"I came out of that delivery room with more respect for my wife than I ever had for her.

"And if that isn't enough, as soon as my son was born, the nurses started sticking tubes up his nose, down his throat, and started sucking all this fluid out to clear his lungs. . . . This only went on for a few minutes, but I mean he was just *born*. I wondered if he was going to make it. Turns out this is routine stuff for them, but it was so *invasive*, so fast. And it was out of our control."

Pain, blood, and loss of control—these are the fears of new fathers who have done their homework as nineties dads. But by learning all they can about childbirth and delivery procedures, male partners can put those fears into perspective even if they can't erase them. After taking childbirth classes men may realize they *can* help do something about their partner's pain, and they *can* do something about a feeling of loss of control in the delivery room. The bleeding, however, remains beyond a male partner's control. "There's still a segment of men who are afraid to be in the room during the delivery," says Dr. Albert George Thomas, a professor of obstetrics and gynecology at Mount Sinai Medical Center in New York City. "So I make sure to ask early on in the pregnancy whether a husband or partner will want to be there for the delivery, and whether they're going to take [childbirth] classes.

"Classes can help them with what to expect, because a lot of men worry about their wives losing too much blood during delivery," Thomas says. "They aren't aware that the mother has produced and 'stored' extra blood for this purpose. And they don't realize that it's not all blood. A lot of the fluid that's lost is water, or water tinged with blood. But it's not all fear on the men's part either. A lot of my patients are working-class, and they're so busy trying to make the next dime that they may not both have time for childbirth classes."

The unfortunate aspect of this, Thomas says, is that if a husband is not willing or able to be with his wife during childbirth, it may make the delivery harder on her. "It's not just a matter of him getting her a glass of ice chips to suck on or holding her hand," he says. "It's that he knows the woman better than anyone else in the room." This aspect of what the male partner can contribute to the delivery team during childbirth is often overlooked. He *knows* the mother; he knows her body and mind. His knowledge and presence can be his most helpful contribution of all.

It's hard to believe that hospitals have only allowed men to be with their wives during childbirth since the mid-1970s. Yet since that time countless fathers have described their presence at their first child's birth as the most exciting day of their lives. It may not be easy of course (or pretty, for that matter), to see your wife or partner in so much pain surrounded by a team of near-strangers. But think of how it used to be: A father didn't see *any* of this, including the birth of his child. "One thing that concerns a lot of fathers is that they don't want the doctors or the delivery to hurt her," says Margaret Truesdale, R.N., the childbirth educator from Boston.

"When I started teaching about childbirth," Truesdale says, referring to the late 1960s, "I remember a man saying, 'In the old days they didn't do all this. A woman would go out into the fields, have a baby, then go back to work.' He was talking about how all this education was a nuisance. But I also remember another man in the class saying, 'They died young all those years ago, too, didn't they?'"

THE STAGES OF LABOR

The first stage of labor begins officially when contractions of the uterus start to dilate (open) the cervix. Stimulated by the hormone oxytocin, the cervix dilates a bit even before a woman is aware it's occurring. A "show" is the other typical biomarker of labor, wherein the mucous plug—a sticky, pink discharge—is loosened and dislodged out of the cervix as the cervix begins to stretch. The contractions occur every fifteen to twenty minutes at first, then increase in strength and frequency as labor continues.

The contractions, which are generally painful at this stage, force the cervix to open to a width of about 4 or 5 centimeters (about 1.6 to 2 inches wide). It is now considered half dilated. Full dilation is at 10 centimeters, or about 4 inches across, approximately the size of a man's fist. For first pregnancies the entire first stage of labor often lasts thirteen or fourteen hours, which is why first-time expectant fathers don't really need to worry about getting stuck in traffic en route to the hospital.

By this time (and sometimes sooner), the amniotic fluid, or bag of waters, breaks, which then gushes out of the birth canal. This in turn causes labor to speed up on two fronts: The baby's head presses down harder on the cervix (now lacking its fluid-and-membrane cushion); and the hormone prostaglandin floods the bloodstream, further inducing contractions.

The next stage, the transition stage of labor, is usually described as the toughest for a woman to endure. By this point the baby's head has moved down the birth canal, and the contractions come quickly in waves. A woman will feel confused, because she'll have an urge to bear down, to push, and yet the delivery staff may urge her not to, until her cervix is judged *fully* dilated. Nausea can also set in. Some women will become frustrated and say they don't want to be touched by anyone at this stage, because of their pain and mixed feelings. Some turn on their partners in anger.

Looking back, Robin P. says that during labor her husband, John, was both supportive and available, yet maybe even too much "in charge." "He was counting and helping me breathe, and he would slow down his counting so that I could bear down harder, push longer. He wanted to be the *best* coach, and he was great. I had a real good labor nurse, and he really worked well with her. He kept me real cool, with cold compresses, ice chips, and his voice. The only thing is, maybe he could have paid a little more attention to me . . . and less to the directions, to the role he was playing."

Paula K. says, "I feel indebted to my husband for the rest of my life, for what he did for me during labor. I couldn't have done it without him. I was so *vulnerable*. I mean, you've never been in pain like that in your life. At one point during early labor I actually got out of the bed and tried to leave the hospital. He said,

'Whoah! Where are you going?' I said, 'I've got to get out of here.' They finally gave me an epidural [anesthetic] and I got some relief."

The best advice doctors can sometimes give to partners during transition is to remain supportive and wait it out—it is usually relatively short, between five minutes and an hour.[7]

THE SECOND STAGE OF LABOR

The second stage of labor is when the baby is born. It is marked by harder, lower contractions, in which the mother feels *forced* to bear down. She is helping to push the baby through the birth canal now, with the cervix fully dilated, as the contractions come every one to two minutes, and last about sixty seconds each.

Guided by the muscles of the pelvis, the baby's head is pushed first (in most births) under the front pelvic bone and through the vagina, at an angle that presents the narrowest width for delivery. In breech births the baby's feet or behind enter the birth canal first. Sometimes these breech births can be delivered vaginally; other times a cesarean section is required. This is a surgical procedure in which an incision is made in the mother's abdomen and the baby is actually lifted out of the uterus. (It is also performed when babies are unusually large, when mothers are known to have sexually transmitted diseases or other medical problems, and in cases when the baby shows signs of distress.)

During a vaginal birth that is not a breech, the baby's head will emerge slightly from the vulva, then often recede, frustratingly, between contractions. The muscles of the pelvic floor and the vulva are active now, pushing along with the uterus to move the baby's head and shoulders—the largest body parts first—out of the birth canal. This allows the rest of the baby's body to slide out with less effort. The second stage of labor, start to finish, typically lasts thirty minutes to an hour (with first births sometimes longer).

For the statistically minded, it may help to know that during second-stage labor a first-time mother spends an average of fifty-seven minutes pushing out her baby, while a second-time mother averages just eighteen minutes.[8] It is during this stage that a couple, often led by the male partner, puts its childbirth education to the test. Regular, rhythmic breathing patterns of the Lamaze method, or similar stress-management and pushing techniques of the (newer) Bradley method go a long way toward distracting a woman from her labor pain. Both techniques aid the mother and delivery team in minimizing the chances of complications. And in both, the woman's partner or "coach" plays an essential role.

After the birth, though seldom during it, new mothers give their partners high marks for every kind of support—emotional, physical, moral, even spiritual. This is your reward as a birthing partner—if you need one.

THE EPISIOTOMY QUESTION

Throughout the pregnancy you may often wonder exactly how a seven-pound baby will actually fit through and emerge from the vagina. Sometimes it can't, without the aid of an episiotomy, a small incision made by the doctor during second-stage labor. And while episiotomies are done almost routinely—in nearly two-thirds of all births in the United States today—there is great debate over whether they are needed so often. The incision, usually between one and a half to two inches long, is made along the perineum, from the bottom of the vaginal opening toward the anus, in order to prevent irregular tearing of the membranes and vagina. It requires a local anesthetic and numerous stitches to close it, but obstetricians often assure first-time mothers that episiotomy is the second most common surgical procedure in the United States, next to the cutting of the umbilical cord.

There is no right or wrong answer before a birth as to whether a woman will need an episiotomy. Couples are urged to discuss their fears and requests with their doctor *well before the birth*, so they won't have to make a split-second decision in the delivery room. Some doctors do episiotomies 90 percent of the time, some only 10 percent of the time. A couple can (and many do) request that one not be done unless absolutely necessary. But it should be noted that painful though the healing process can be during recovery, it may reduce discomfort over the long term in many cases and can save a baby from dangerous distress.

"I have strong opinions on whether men should have a say in matters like this," says Paula K. "He is entitled to his position, he has a right to it. But he doesn't have the right to dictate to me whether I should have an episiotomy, or whether the delivery should be 'drug-free.' It's something that can't be foreseen. It's my body. I had an episiotomy on doctor's orders and I tore anyway." Doctors point out, in cases like Paula's, that she may have suffered a more dangerous tear if she hadn't had the episiotomy.

A final note on a sensitive subject: If a doctor suggests that an episiotomy will improve a couple's sex life by "making her tighter when I sew her up," don't believe it. In fact intercourse is oftentimes painful long after an episiotomy, due to the delicate nature of the muscles and skin of the perineum. Sutures made too tight here may only add to the recovery time and potential for pain. The question should not be one of "tightness" but one of assuring safe delivery of the baby and minimizing the mother's tissue damage.

THE THIRD STAGE OF LABOR

The easiest and most comfortable stage of labor is stage three, which begins at delivery of the baby and lasts through delivery of the placenta, or afterbirth. This stage, after the grueling hours of labor and months of pregnancy, typically lasts from a few minutes to half an hour.

Since the uterus is almost empty now, the final contractions of childbirth quickly shrink it as the placenta is sloughed away from its inner wall. In essence the uterus is attempting to close up blood vessels that had nourished the fetus for so long. The doctor may massage the mother's abdomen and tug gently on the umbilical cord that remains (to hasten the afterbirth), and a drug that mimics oxytocin is also sometimes used to speed the process and minimize bleeding.

The irony here is that after all the work of delivering a baby, a mother may have mixed emotions at just the point one would expect her to be giddy with delight. A father too. There is no more powerful moment, first-time parents often say, than when a pink, crinkly, healthy baby is laid gently on the exhausted mother's chest. It's time for smiles, and tears. Oddly, though, the tears of joy are often accompanied by a simultaneous wish on the part of the mother *to be left alone*. She may feel an urgent need to recover from all the physical work she's just done. Some mothers even exhibit a kind of shock reaction, replete with chills, chattering teeth, and severe trembling. But this, too, subsides quickly as the body recovers from the shock of the new. Goodbye, pregnancy. Hello, postpartum period.

WHAT MEN CAN DO

In the relatively recent history of husbands joining their wives in the delivery room, many a first-time father has wished for a simple checklist he could use to help his partner through labor. Faced with mounds of childbirth books and maternity magazines, men have longed for something leaner. Wouldn't that make sense? The editors of *Childbirth* magazine conferred and published the following list in the 1990 issue of their annual magazine. This list isn't meant to supplant six weeks of prepared-childbirth classes; it is, however, up-to-date and useful. During labor a male partner can:

1. Tell his partner how much he loves her, how well she's doing; hug and kiss her a lot.
2. Help her to change positions. Check that she urinates about once per hour. Walk with her around the room or hospital halls. Help her to squat and push when she needs to.
3. Stroke, massage, and grip tense areas of her body. Remind her gently to let go of tension, but don't give orders to her to "relax."
4. Apply hot compresses or a hot-water bottle as she wishes; and help her with a shower or warm bath if time allows (and if such facilities are available).
5. Take charge if she gets discouraged, reminding her to take the contractions one at a time. Also remind her that she did really well "growing" the baby all these months and that her body knows what to do now as well. (If she says she can't do it anymore, you can tell her she can and *is* doing it and that you're going to help her make it through.)
6. Apply a cool cloth to her forehead or sponge her off.
7. Bring her a snack or drink, or spoon ice chips into her mouth a bit at a time.
8. Establish eye contact and maintain it. (If she tenses up too rigidly and closes her eyes, you can tell her to open them and fixate on your eyes for a moment.)
9. Help her to breathe rhythmically by breathing along with her. Remind her to "breathe away" tension.
10. Count off fifteen-second intervals during contractions, reminding her when they are at the halfway point and thus ready to fade in intensity.

Throughout labor, a man can do a lot for his partner by acting as her advocate. With some advance planning and preparation he may be able to make her delivery less stressful by speaking up for her and being assertive. For example, the questions of medication during delivery can and should be discussed thoroughly beforehand by the couple and the doctor. During labor, if the mother is not in a position to argue with the hospital staff, her partner can voice her requests for her. The more contact a partner has had with his wife's delivery team prior to labor, the smoother these interactions will be when it counts.

BREAST-FEEDING AND THINKING ANEW ABOUT BREASTS

Once the baby is born, the first contact you may witness, often while still in the delivery room, arises from the baby's urge to suckle a breast. Contrary to what first-time fathers may think, this isn't all about hunger. It's a reflex action on the baby's part, and it encourages a number of changes in the mother's body.

One of these is, of course, lactation, the milk-producing action of the breasts. Another change takes place in the mother's pituitary gland. The act of suckling encourages the production of the hormones oxytocin and prolactin, which in turn help shrink the uterus back to its original size and stimulate the milk glands to push milk along through the reservoirs and milk ducts and out through the nipples. For the first couple of days colostrum, a nutrient-laden substance, is produced; breast milk appears in most cases by the third day after delivery. Some women feel acute, though quickly passing pain, when their milk "comes in."

As for the breasts themselves, they produce as much milk as the baby needs. They also supply nutrients and antibodies (to protect the newborn against infection) of the highest order. Breasts may become sore, however, from the combination of their swollen size and the baby's sucking of the nipples. Many women give up breast-feeding after a few weeks or months because of the enormous time constraints involved—often ten or more feedings per day. Others combine breast-feeding with bottle-formula, which offers a father a chance to get more intimately involved with feeding his newborn child.

Paralleling the rise of fathers in delivery rooms, the number of women who have chosen to breast-feed has climbed steadily in recent years. Among mothers today two-thirds opt to breast-feed their infants, despite the high incidence of women in the work force. As recently as 1970 only one mother in four nursed her newborn.[9]

Among the unexpected physical reactions reported by mothers breast-feeding for the first time are warm, sensual, quivering feelings that flow as the baby suckles a breast. Some women say they occasionally have orgasms while nursing. While this may both shock and please the woman, it can be unsettling for a father who feels he is left out of the picture, especially if he is unfamiliar with the physiological facts of breast-feeding.

One first-time father I interviewed reported a breast-feeding-bonding experience with a twist. One night, he said, his wife was having trouble "letting down" the milk in her breasts to pump and store for future feedings. She told her husband about it while their three-month-old daughter was asleep. He approached his wife, knelt down, and began to gently suck her right nipple for a minute or two. It wasn't in the baby books they'd read, but it worked. They undoubtedly aren't the first couple to try such a procedure, but they felt as if they were: it was new *to them*. It was also a little unsettling, he said. "Even though I've been playing with her breasts for seven years, it felt sort of 'illegal' because she's a new mother and all. We didn't know what to feel." One thing's for sure, they felt like parents.

SEX AND PREGNANCY

While men like to joke from time to time about the evaporation of their sex lives during and after pregnancy, many couples find there's both humor and frustration in dealing with "pregnant sex."

"You know, you get very horny when you're pregnant," Paula K. says. "And if you multiply those feelings by ten, to cover the orgasms you supposedly have everyday in your sleep, it can be a pretty wild time. But there's another thing men should know: I absolutely did not want my breasts touched at all. I mean, they *hurt*. The first three months I was pregnant, even the wind blowing on me would hurt. At that point I realized my breasts belonged to 'the baby.' And none of this is a big deal if you say it up front."

"There were a couple of times [during my pregnancy] when I was horny," says Colleen H. "But it didn't surprise me when it happened because I was so overread on the subject. I'd read five million books, so I had come to the conclusion that any way I feel about sex during pregnancy is totally acceptable. Some books say women get very horny; others say some women lose sexual desire totally during those nine months. There is *no* norm, because in the end nothing about anybody else's experience with sex means anything to your own." When they did have intercourse, the pregnant Colleen and her husband used side-by-side and rear-entry positions, and they didn't "bounce around" as much as they had before she was pregnant. But they both had orgasms, and they weren't afraid of sex during these months.

"Early on," adds Colleen, "sometimes at the slightest [sexual] stimulation, you get a letdown [of milk]—in bed! Now, I've heard some guys get turned on by this, but frankly I don't think lying in a pool of milk is sexy. Sometimes you just want to say, 'Later. I'm leaky, stay the hell away.' "

"I had a lot more sex during my second pregnancy than my first," says Robin P., "but I think part of that is because my second husband is a lot more sexual than my first. The second time I had sex up until my eighth or ninth month. I have to say, though, it does get awkward toward the end, because you're so big you can't really move much. My doctor said, 'You can have sex [toward the end of the pregnancy], but don't have enemas.' " This last caveat was to guard against jump-starting labor prematurely.

Interestingly, researchers have uncovered reports of women (and men) who find sex during even late stages of pregnancy incredibly arousing, sometimes resulting in multiple orgasms for women who don't normally experience them.[10]

In time men who use the weeks of pregnancy as a kind of graduate school in female anatomy may find it easier to talk about sex and reproductive health than they ever did before. Pregnancy is, after all, a natural time for partners to talk about physically intimate matters, no matter how shy they may have been about these things before. And ironically, even while a couple may not have sex for weeks at a time, the pregnancy that may be keeping them physically apart can bring them psychologically closer. Sexual feelings—new ones—naturally emerge, and a doctor or childbirth educator (even unintentionally) can act as a bridge between the partners.

"They [men] also want to know, 'Can we have intercourse while she's pregnant?' " Margaret Truesdale, R.N., says. "When I tell them that it's an old wives' tale to stop having sex six weeks before the baby is due, when I say yes, that comforts them. What we're finding is that there are no real restrictions on sex during pregnancy—as long as care is taken."

"With my first baby," says Sheila B., thirty-two, "my doctor wanted my husband and me to have sex all the way to the end of the pregnancy. 'It's good for you,' he said. And even after the baby was born, he didn't think we had to stop six weeks before [the birth]—and wait six weeks to start up again. 'You'll heal in three days,' he said. 'Just be careful.' "

"In the ninth month, we weren't having sex anymore." Paula says. "From the seventh month on, I was very cautious about having sex because I didn't want to have any more orgasms that could trigger labor. I know it's unlikely that would happen, but I didn't even want the *possibility*. Before that I would just get on top or over on my side, because you can't do the missionary position."

As for the facts on the lesser-sex side, some women find sex during pregnancy not only unstimulating but uncomfortable. Many women have a decreased sex drive early in their pregnancy and simply do not want to be fondled. Similarly, they may feel uncomfortable with their tender breasts and nipples or with their slightly swollen vaginal lips. Or they may be suffering from morning sickness and (naggingly real) headaches. Men who know this up front may avoid feelings of rejection later on.

"In terms of what I'd tell men about this," Colleen says, "I'd say, 'Let patience be your watchword.' Because the few times during my pregnancy when I remember *really* being in the mood for sex, I could not have imagined anything worse than someone being pushy. I remember thinking, 'You don't understand; I'm a *tank*. You don't understand the kind of pain I'm in. It's just really tough. It's just hard to get comfortable, even if the sex [intercourse] itself doesn't hurt."

POSTPARTUM LOVEMAKING

After birth a new set of sexual guidelines and feelings—again wide-ranging—comes into play. From the mother's perspective, hormonal changes actually suppress her sex drive during the postpartum period. Decreased estrogen levels are the most common reason, which may also cause bouts of vaginal dryness for weeks after delivery. Likewise the postpartum depression many couples hear about isn't another old wives' tale. It's physiological fact, one that occurs in 3 to 23 percent of all women.[11]

Another physiological fact to consider is that after childbirth, a woman's vagina and pelvic-floor muscles need time to heal. In cases where an episiotomy was performed, scar tissue will form around the stitches, resulting in the need for extra-careful love-making for weeks in some cases, months in others. In general, couples often resume sexual activity within four to six weeks, with a few tentative steps.

While some women heal more quickly than others, it's important for both partners to talk about and acknowledge the pain that persists. Otherwise, passive, mechanical sex, or even resentment on the part of the new mother, may follow. Deep penetration during intercourse, for instance, may be off limits for some couples for months. For others it may not be a problem.

"The best explanation I can give men," says Colleen, "about how it feels after giving birth [vaginally], is something a friend of mine told me: 'You hurt from stem to stern.' What I remember about it was that, at one point, during the first week after I had Laura, I was in pain and I was wondering, 'Is it my stitches that hurt? Or . . . is it my hemorrhoids?' Then I thought, 'Why am I even *trying* to figure this *out*? Does it matter?'

"After you give birth, you don't want it to hurt anymore, but it's kind of like a muscle," Colleen says of the postpartum vagina. "It only gets better if you *use* it. I remember asking a friend of mine whose baby was six months older than Laura how long it took before it didn't hurt anymore to have sex after her delivery. 'It *still* hurts,' she said."

"Yep," Robin says, "you do get stretched out [vaginally] during delivery. Especially after an eight-pounder's been shoved through there. When I told John, 'I'm a little larger than I was,' he said, 'Yeah, I noticed a little bit.'"

From a father's point of view, the changes he feels regarding postpartum sex may be far-reaching. One writer said it bluntly in *American Baby* magazine: "Getting used to the changes in your sex life—everything from the frequency to the style of your lovemaking—can be one of the hardest parts of new fatherhood."[12]

Although they've always heard it's the mother who won't want sex after childbirth, many men notice a lack of desire for sex that they have trouble explaining. (And they often keep it hidden, out of fear.) Doctors believe a lot of these cases occur because men cannot easily reconcile the physical trauma and function of childbirth with the more sexual side of the female sex organs.

As Henry Edwards, M.D., psychiatrist from Washington, D.C., told me in an interview, some men, whether or not they are highly educated, simply do not want to get "too involved" with their wives' or partners' reproductive health. They would prefer to leave it to the doctors. And it's not that these men are necessarily squeamish. No, Edwards thinks it has more to do with *certain* men's predilection for thinking of their partner's body as a kind of sex object. Feminists and others may view this as small-minded or sexist, but it remains part of the male psyche that presents itself—warts and all—in couples' therapy sessions.

Angela F., thirty-seven, a Connecticut mother of a two-year-old, has had personal experience with this. Her husband joined her in the delivery room when she gave birth to a nine-and-a-half-pound baby, and in retrospect she wishes he wouldn't have seen it all from quite so close. "Maybe men shouldn't be in the delivery room," she says, going against a tide that has risen since 1970 when Dr. Fernand Lamaze published *Painless Childbirth: The Lamaze Method*. She continues to refer to her own indecorous labor as "the construction site," and she bemoans the fact that her husband didn't want to have sex with her for six months after their baby's birth. "I finally asked him why," she says, "because it was clear he wasn't going to bring it up. He complained about my breast-feeding, about how there were milk spots all over, stains on the sheets, and that he didn't find me as appealing as before."

Not only was Angela upset by her husband's answer, she was angry that she had to do the asking. That *she* was responsible for "healing" this sexual rift that was caused in part by the physical brutality of a difficult childbirth. Was all this fair? What men can learn from Angela's experiences has as much to do with sex and marriage as it does with childbirth. Even before she was pregnant, Angela felt she was burdened by being in charge of the couple's sex life. She still is. Having the baby didn't change the ways they dealt with sex or their communication, which isn't surprising. Pregnancy doesn't "fix" problems like this in a relationship, just as it doesn't really cause them. In this case it exacerbated them by magnifying them. And unfortunately it caught Angela and her husband unprepared for the unease that would follow.

When couples are aware of the potential problems associated with sex and pregnancy, however, they can shed their fears in each other's company and move on. And as we've seen in this chapter, expectant parents may find a host of sexual pleasures along the way if they know where to look: Oftentimes experimenting with new positions of intercourse, such as rear entry, results in a lifelong change of sexual habits. Many women find they enjoy the increased fondling that occurs when their male partners' hands are freed up from their weight-bearing role in the missionary position. Other couples say they were actually surprised at the sexual pleasure they experienced in the last trimester, according to Elisabeth Bing, a noted childbirth educator and author of *Making Love During Pregnancy*.

"Frequently pregnant women have an unusually strong desire for sex," Bing says. "Many report that they first experienced orgasm at that time [the last three months]." The reason? Well, it *could* be the increased attention and sensitivity on the part of the male partner. But it could also be that the increased blood flow to and through the pelvic area during pregnancy can make a woman's genitals just that much more sensitive, more responsive, to touch and to other sensual pleasures.

CHAPTER 11

FINAL THOUGHTS:

WHAT WOMEN WISH

MEN KNEW

Lynne M., a single twenty-eight-year-old living outside of Boston, had a boyfriend who was a selfish lover: On a typical night he'd climb on top, have an orgasm in a hurry, then pull away and go to sleep. Sometimes he'd tell her how good it felt before he drifted off. She would lie next to him, silent and empty. And sad. When Lynne complained about the pattern to a friend, her friend told her to talk to her boyfriend instead.

It was only then that Lynne recognized the irony of her situation: An extremely articulate, outgoing person, she didn't feel comfortable enough to *talk* with him about anything intimate, yet she was sleeping with him two or three times a week. Ultimately she did talk with him, and things improved a bit in bed before they broke up. But her initial response—her fear of making waves, "threatening" the relationship, or challenging a fragile male ego—isn't unique. For many it's the norm.

Throughout the course of my research for this book the sobering refrain among women has been, "Why can't men just understand that . . . ?" about everything from etiquette to intimacy to hormones. Well, I often wondered, why can't women tell them? Jocelyn W., someone I would not describe as shy, hints at one of the possible reasons: "It's easier sometimes to fake an orgasm than it is to explain to somebody what you want." It's not that Jocelyn, twenty-seven, doesn't enjoy orgasms. It's more that she puts her needs to have an intact relationship ahead of her sexual ones (at least for now). And unlike Lynne, Jocelyn isn't afraid to talk about sex with her partners. She merely waits, she says, until she thinks the relationship is on solid ground before broaching the subject. Till then she is content (if not happy) either to wait things out or to exit the relationship altogether.

Then there's Janice C., thirty-five, a married artist, who could tell *me* her erotic fantasies but couldn't tell them to her husband. "I would feel silly or inhibited," she explained. But that's not getting her—or the rest of us—anywhere.

Maybe the fact that I was a nonthreatening stranger uninvolved in their lives made it easier for many women to reveal their secrets or wishes to me. Without the risk of rejection, confrontation, or abandonment, women could tell me things they didn't feel free to discuss with their husbands, lovers, boyfriends, and exes. So, toward the end of our interviews I asked them, "If you could tell men (or your man) one thing about your body or yourself that hasn't gotten through, what would it be? What do you wish men knew?"

"Sex and emotions are profoundly connected."

"I need to trust someone before I can feel any semblance of security being with that man," says Rachel B., a twenty-three-year-old single Chicagoan. And trust—much less security—isn't easy to come by these days.

In the same vein, although Saundra S., twenty-seven, of New York City, loves and trusts her husband, she told me it's frustrating that she "can't shift gears" the way he can. She needs to be emotionally ready before she can really make love. "I think my husband already knows everything about my body," she says. "But I wish he could understand that if I have a lot of things on my mind—a busy day at work or whatever—that I would rather he let me unwind before he makes a pass at me. I'm more receptive to his advances after I've resolved my problems." It turns out Saundra is wrong about one thing: She says her husband "knows everything" about her body, but he obviously falls short when it comes to one significant part—her mind.

"My attitude has changed recently," says Adrian P., thirty-six, a divorced mother of one from Denver, and she says it's not due to the fear of AIDS. "Most of my relationships have been physical early on, where I would have sex by the second date. Now I want the emotional side to develop first before I have any physical relations. In my current relationship we see each other a lot and we don't have sex on every date. My partner is understanding. He listened to what I had to say and said, 'I know what you need—lots of hugs.' "

Deborah M., twenty-five, of New York City, was infuriated because her sometime lover didn't always call her the morning after they'd spent the night together. "Finally I just told him he had to call me or I couldn't sleep with him anymore. It didn't end, for me, with the sex. I needed to know it had to be *my* body and not just any body. I needed to feel there was a connection more than he did." Setting aside the so-called sexual revolutionary mores, most women said they couldn't just have sex. They wanted, and needed, to "make love."

Then, of course, there were a few exceptions. "Sometimes," says Roxanne F., twenty-five, from Arlington, Virginia, "you *do* just want to have sex . . . like men do. They don't seem to know that that's how we think sometimes too. They think it's something that's deeper for us. It isn't always."

Given the wide variety of experience and preferences women expressed, it's surprising to find that women were at all consistent in what they wanted men to know about their sexual selves. But there were some recurring themes. Such as . . . fondling, foreplay, and afterplay.

"What I would like more of but I don't request because I feel slightly silly or inhibited is an all-over body massage," says Janice C., of New York, "something done in a teasing, titillating way, that involved a lot of touching, prolonging the massage and slowly building up to massaging my genital area. That would be really arousing."

Faye R., twenty-eight and from Connecticut, agrees. "Men should fondle more—hair, hands, back—and not spend so much time on the breasts. Especially before sex." In a way it's ironic that Faye said the word *sex* when she meant to say *intercourse*. For she clearly wants the proportion of sex versus intercourse to shift in the direction of more foreplay and more varied physical touching. "If women aren't sufficiently aroused," she adds, "it won't be as good. And this is easy to do: Rub the clitoris. But many men either don't realize it or find this unpleasant, which in turn makes women feel bad about themselves."

"Guys still think we like it when they are rough and forceful with their fingers," says Paige A., twenty, a college student from Athens, Georgia. "I like them to be gentle and caring." A sense of urgency, of rushing through the "preliminaries," makes sex less enjoyable for Paige, who nonetheless remains both impressionable and hopeful.

On a similar note, Callie K., twenty-eight, of Albuquerque, New Mexico, says, "I think a lot of men still need to learn that women are just more sensitive, physically, than they are." When Callie talks about sensitivity, she is talking about two different things: the actual pressure men apply with their hands, fingers, and mouths to various parts of women's bodies and also the awareness men have in regard to reading their partners' overall desires.

Sue P., forty-two, a widow living outside Milwaukee, Wisconsin, says, "Men I've had sex with have tended either to 'attack' with too much vigor—the more pressure the better—or they've approached me too timidly, as if they were afraid of hurting me. When I try to help them, most of the time they feel threatened and then they retreat. Many have admitted not wanting to know more about women's bodies. It's as if it's all too complicated for them, or else they *think* they know enough to get by (or that they know it *all*). I think the male ego still gets in the way of even the most confident men, when it comes to sex and women."

Sue's wish to "educate" her men about how she likes to be touched brings up an even broader question of how to talk with a lover without hurting his or her feelings. In her case she expects that men who aren't confident about their sexual selves will balk at receiving instructions from their lovers, yet she seems surprised to find that even the more confident men take refuge and hide behind their egos. She has been with several men who tell her they want to please her, but who then revert to their old behaviors. They aren't always being selfish, she says, but merely resistant to admitting their past "mistakes." One way around this impasse is for men to acknowledge the individuality of women's sexual preferences and the fact that what pleases one partner may turn off another. No matter how well the women you've been with may have taught you, there are no fail-safe rules about female sexual pleasure—except for the rule that says, "Each woman wants to be caressed individually."

Michael Castleman, a health educator and writer from northern California, wrote in his book, *Sexual Solutions*, that one of the major problems men have with sex today is a distorted focus on foreplay. By calling it *foreplay*, in fact, Castleman says, we tend to place too much importance on the act of intercourse (since foreplay implies that what comes later is what we're really waiting for). Along the same lines, Castleman isn't enamored of the word *afterplay*. Instead he introduces the notion of "loveplay," as the kind of touching, caressing, and overall stimulation two lovers enjoy before, after, or *instead* of intercourse, depending on their moods. And while the word hasn't exactly caught on in the sexological community, it's worth remembering the next time you think about why we do what we do in bed.

"Beyond a woman's mouth and her vagina," says Catherine S., thirty-eight, "I think men think a woman has three other erogenous zones: two nipples and a clitoris. So, after the kissing, they do a little with the nipples and the clit, then move on to screwing. It's so *predictable* and so *boring*! They forget the massive areas of skin—neck, back, stomach, legs." And of course their minds.

"If only men understood our bodies better."

On this point the chorus of women's voices I heard may not have been loud, but it certainly was clear. "Let's face it," says Lori E., twenty-nine, a married attorney. "In order for a man and a woman to be sexually compatible, the man needs to have a general working knowledge of her erogenous zones. Perhaps knowledge will increase sensitivity."

"If men knew more about women's bodies," says Robin G., twenty-eight and married, "it would relieve a lot of the frustration that we as couples face during sex. I think that my husband's inability to satisfy me sometimes comes not from his lack of desire but from his lack of knowledge. . . . You can't understand and deal with what you don't know."

Jocelyn W., twenty-seven, adds, "Men think that if a woman has an orgasm, they've 'done their job.' That's not true."

"I have a very low sex drive, and my boyfriend knows that," says Amy H., twenty-four, a law student from Berkeley, California, "but it's really a matter of appreciating it. He acts like he's seventeen years old," Amy says, clearly frustrated. "I wish that he would recognize the difference between men and women and their drives." (She mentions this sex-drive difference as a given, although it is still being debated.) "Most women I know are not that keen on having sex every single night," she adds, "unless they're really concerned about the guy—and feel like they've got to keep someone around. I wish that my boyfriend would realize that if I don't want to have sex some night, it's not an indication that I don't find him attractive or that he doesn't turn me on.

"Every time I *do* have sex, I think, 'Why don't I do this more often?' But it's just not a major part of my life, and I think guys miss that. Sometimes I think guys' entire lives are about getting laid."

Janice C., thirty-five, says, "It seems easier to get to know a man's body. They are so much more easily aroused than women. My husband once told me that if a *monkey* touched his dick, he would get a hard-on. I think that if men knew more about women's bodies and the hormonal changes we go through, they would be more supportive and understanding. Like when a woman is yelling at the top of her lungs, it would be easier for a partner to stay calm and not take it personally. Fights wouldn't escalate."

"I wish men knew more not just about women's bodies," says Betsy R., "but about *women*." As a health care worker who deals every day with the care of the physiological self, she would prefer it if men spent as much (or more) time assessing the psychological selves of their female partners as they do the sexual ones.

Jill C., thirty-three and married, says, "I wish men had the interest to *want* to understand more about our bodies."

Judy W., thirty-six, has very specific ideas about what men should know. "I wish men could understand the changes I go through during the month," says Judy. "My PMS [premenstrual syndrome] symptoms begin about ten days before I get my period. I wish men could understand that I'm not unpleasant because I have a bad attitude but that my irritability has a physiological basis. I feel achy, anxious, and I have a desire to be alone and read or sleep.

"My last husband would notice my mood swings and say, 'Oh, Christ, she's having her period again,' " she says. "He would make a lot of sarcastic, negative remarks. I don't think men actually try to understand how a woman may be feeling during her period or if she has PMS."

"The one thing I wish," says Liza R., twenty-one, a college student in Providence, Rhode Island, "is that men wouldn't be so squeamish talking about when a woman gets her period. I don't think guys have a clue as to how it feels for us to be bleeding like that. Guys should just accept that this is a fact of life, and women go through it every month. If you want to be a part of their lives, well, it happens, and you can't expect a woman not to talk about it. It's there for a fifth to a quarter of her life."

Not only do women's bodies and feelings change during the course of the month, but, as Gwen R., thirty-two, anticipates, they change over time. She says: "I would ask my husband to prepare himself to accept the changes my body will be going through if and when I get pregnant and as I age. I haven't been pregnant yet, so it's uncharted territory. And I don't really think men are very accepting of women's aging. I know several men who divorced their wives to marry younger women. My history of anorexia has something to do with my anxiety; I'm worried that I'm going to be twice as big as my husband."

Suzanne L., thirty-five and married, has already gone through some physical changes. "My breasts used to be the most eroge-nous part of my body, but ever since I nursed my daughter, my breasts have lost a lot of their sensitivity. Now I'm in the process of trying to find a new erogenous zone. I need to find a new way to get turned on." For Suzanne some things also remain the same. "I'd like to reenact some of the more erotic sexual experi-ences of my youth with my husband, but I think it would hurt his feelings. I was very adventurous in high school and college: I like having sex in semipublic places, where there's some danger in being discovered. My husband isn't really one to do anything where you can get caught."

What might seem like an overwhelming task—understanding a woman's body every day of the month, every year of her life—is actually a finite task, according to Mary C., twenty-six. She says, "Some things should be private. In general, men should know the *basics* of woman's reproductive parts, but nothing's worse than a know-it-all male telling you what *your* body is doing."

"Women often crave affection more than sex; many say they'll settle for consideration."

Randi H., twenty-five, a single New Yorker, says, "Do you know how *cute* it is for a guy just to kiss you?" The message Randi wants to convey to the men in her life is that *affection counts*—maybe more so than the grander, typically sexy gesture.

"I want a man to be considerate, but I don't want to be smothered," says Catherine S., thirty-eight. "I just want him to do what he says he'll do: If he says he'll call, he should call."

"There's this guy I'm seeing now," says Candace, twenty-four, of Long Island, New York, "whom I just started seeing a few weeks ago. He called me up yesterday and said, 'I just wanted you to know that I'm thinking warm thoughts about you.' I couldn't *wait* to see him."

When it comes to relationships and affection, Connie M., thirty-four, a married mother of three, has a more sweeping, perceptive perspective: "Women's expectations of men are so low, really," she says. "If [my husband] Jeff could pick up on that, it would be great. It's strictly psychology, really." Connie also believes that it's not all that difficult for her husband—or for other husbands—to break through to a higher level.

"I say to him, 'It's the little things that make me like you.' It's not birthdays that are important, it's day-to-day living . . . when you think he's doing nice things for you because he *likes* you, not because he loves you!" A lot of men may find this compelling: a woman who gets turned on more by "like" than "love," who's looking for her man's affection because somehow, after ten years of marriage, it feels to her more honest, more genuine.

"Women want to feel powerful—and unique—and men can help."

On a clear summer night in the French Riviera, on the last concert stop of her 1990 "Blond Ambition" world tour, Madonna, the American diva of rock musical choreography, looked out at her audience, reached down with her right hand, and grabbed her crotch.

"*I'm* the boss here," she said through the space-age headset microphone that enabled her to keep her hands free while performing. The preening, the prancing, the gender-bending garb she wore and then the crotch grab, on cue, were all planned—part of The Show.

Madonna struck a pose; there was something to it. It was a pose favored by macho-striving men of all stripes. And in so doing, she was straddling a blurry gender line, yet she wasn't trying to alienate men. Her gesture added a link in the chain of evolution of how certain women today feel about—or are *supposed* to feel about—their sexuality. More and more, they want to feel openly comfortable with it. All of it.

The way Madonna Louise Ciccone grabbed herself, she made it look like fun. And while she wasn't exactly stimulating herself, she was stimulating more than a little thought. She was saying to men and women, *"The sexual power game is changing—it really is."*

Faye R., twenty-eight, who is single and lives in Connecticut, is not a huge Madonna fan, but she knows what she likes and she, too, likes to wield the sexual power of seduction. The difference is she prefers to perform in one-on-one settings, not before millions. "Men should know that women get turned on when we know *we're* turning someone on!" Faye says. "Also, knowing that someone's efforts to please me are due to his desire to make me happy more than his efforts to impress me makes me feel special, less inhibited, more giving and relaxed."

Marcia A., thirty and single, agrees that the power is in the specifics of what's said and done between two people, irrespective of gender. "If I could tell men one thing about my body, it would be, 'Please, please, tell me what's good about *this* one. Leave other women's bodies out of it. Tell me how you like this *particular* curve—that my ass is perfect. Please don't tell me I have small *but nice* breasts. If men are like women—and I believe they are—in the sense that they get attached to something specific, about me, particularly my smell, they should tell me.

"I wish men knew how easy it was to make a woman like sex with them. Easy. Be into her body, be into getting her off, tell her how great she's making you feel. Tell her you think about her when you're in a meeting or driving somewhere; I swear, she'll keep coming back."

Of course no one person, not even Madonna, can cause a massive shift between the sexes. And still another sexual revolution, if and when it occurs, is almost beside the point. Because men and women want to understand what's happening *now* between the sexes. Not surprisingly, it's unsettled. One year after the "Blond Ambition" tour, a quirky, scholarly book was doing its own dance at the top of the best-seller lists: *You Just Don't Understand: Men and Women in Conversation*, by Deborah Tannen, Ph.D. Not far below was *Iron John: A Book About Men*, by Robert Bly. Why these two? Because at this point in time both sexes crave translations of sorts. Because even in the freewheeling, postmodern, postfeminist, post-first-wave-of-AIDS 1990s, we're still speaking different languages.

If you yourself sense a shift among women or, more to the point, among the thoughts of the woman closest to you, chances are you'll want to react to it in a positive way. You'll also want to know how what's happening at home (or in society) might affect you in the future. These aren't selfish or outrageous male desires; they're reasonable. Nobody wants to play any new power game without having been briefed on the rules.

In short, what's happening between the sexes is a long-awaited realignment of responsibilities and stereotypes, and much of it is for the better. Consider: From the end of the Victorian era through most of the twentieth century, men tended to have (or thought they should have) more of the sexual *experience* coming into a relationship. Women, meanwhile, tended to take responsibility for birth control and for *information* about the couple's sexual health. Women often assumed, then, that their male partners were more "powerful" (by virtue of their experience) in matters of sex, even though this wasn't always so.

In modern relationships sexual power is based on both experience *and* information. So neither partner has an inherent advantage in amassing it. In fact, as we've seen throughout the book, it can be argued that many women, by virtue of their regular gynecological checkups, birth control and pregnancy experiences, and the slew of "relationship" literature aimed at them, can be considered the more sexually (if less physically) powerful partner. Women have also gained sexual power as they've gained more sexual experience at younger ages than their mothers and grandmothers ever had. They've been gaining it for some time now. At last count some 40 percent of young people have had sex by the ninth grade, by about age fourteen, according to the federal Centers for Disease Control.

On the other hand, hundreds of thousands of men recently have learned—by listening to the women in their lives—to explore women more openly, more completely. They've gotten this far by making an effort to secure a base of knowledge and to expand it over time. Which is exactly what millions of women have been busy doing over the past twenty or so years.

Fortunately, relationship experts say, as a shift of sexual power evolves, it won't take anything away from men's or women's sexual selves. "I don't mind giving up power—or whatever you call it," says Laura M., thirty-eight and single, "if it means guys will know how to please me. Or at least ask how." Because every woman is so different, and because their minds and moods and bodies may change at a pace unfamiliar to us, or in ways too subtle for us to detect, sometimes the most we *can* do is to ask. In the long run, it's not technique or terminology, power or experience, that really matters to a woman. It's getting what she wants.

APPENDIX

SURVEY

QUESTIONNAIRE

INTRODUCTORY INFORMATION

FIRST NAME: _____

LAST INITIAL (OPTIONAL): _____

HOME: (STATE OR REGION, E.G., MIDWEST, SOUTH): _____

GENERAL CAREER FIELD: _____

RELIGION (OPTIONAL): _____

MARITAL STATUS: _____ AGE: _____

SEX: FEMALE _____ MALE _____

QUESTION 1

DO YOU THINK MOST WOMEN YOU KNOW ARE COMFORTABLE WITH THEIR BODIES? WHY OR WHY NOT?

_____

_____

_____

QUESTION 2

DO YOU THINK MOST MEN YOU KNOW ARE COMFORTABLE WITH THEIR BODIES? WHY OR WHY NOT?

_____

_____

_____

QUESTION 3

DO YOU WISH MEN KNEW MORE ABOUT WOMEN'S BODIES IN GENERAL? WHY OR WHY NOT? (IF YOU NEED MORE ROOM, PLEASE USE BACK OF FORM.)

_____

_____

_____

QUESTION 4

SPECIFICALLY, IS IT IMPORTANT FOR YOUR SEXUAL PARTNER(S) TO UNDERSTAND HOW FEMALE HORMONES WORK, FROM PUBERTY TO PREGNANCY TO PREMENSTRUAL SYNDROME (PMS) AND BEYOND? WHY OR WHY NOT?

_____

_____

_____

QUESTION 5

ARE YOU TRULY RELAXED WHEN NAKED WITH YOUR (MOST RECENT) PART-
NER OR MATE? DOES HE/SHE SEEM RELAXED WHEN NAKED? WHY OR WHY
NOT? DO YOU USE THE WORDS *VAGINA* AND *PENIS* IN SPEAKING WITH
EACH OTHER?

_____

_____

_____

QUESTION 6

HAS YOUR DATING OR SEXUAL BEHAVIOR CHANGED SINCE YOU'VE
LEARNED MORE ABOUT ACQUIRED IMMUNE DEFICIENCY SYNDROME
(AIDS)? IF SO, HOW?

_____

_____

_____

QUESTION 7

WHAT DO YOU THINK IS THE DIFFERENCE BETWEEN ''GOOD'' AND
''BAD'' SEX?

_____

_____

_____

QUESTION 8

IN *THE HITE REPORT*, PUBLISHED IN 1976, AUTHOR SHERE HITE LISTED
NUMEROUS EXAMPLES OF MEN BEING UNAWARE OF HOW TO STIMULATE A
WOMAN SEXUALLY, OF BEING ''ROUGH'' WITH THEIR HANDS AND FIN-
GERS. DO YOU THINK MEN HAVE GOTTEN ''WISER'' SINCE THEN? WHY?

_____

_____

_____

QUESTION 9

CAN YOU THINK OF A TIME IN WHICH YOU'VE GOTTEN EXCITED SEXUALLY BY MERELY *TALKING* WITH A PARTNER? IF SO, WHEN, AND WHY?

_____

_____

_____

QUESTION 10

HOW IMPORTANT IS LOVE TO YOUR OWN SENSUAL AND SEXUAL PLEA-SURE?

_____

_____

_____

THANK YOU FOR YOUR TIME, CONTRIBUTIONS, AND HONESTY. IF YOU WANT MORE INFORMATION ABOUT THE WORK-IN-PROGRESS, PLEASE WRITE TO:

CURTIS PESMEN
C/O MS. JULIE MERBERG, EDITOR
BALLANTINE BOOKS
201 EAST **50**TH STREET
NEW YORK, NY **10022**

IF YOU WOULD LIKE TO SUGGEST FAMILY, FRIENDS, OR CO-WORKERS FOR PERSONAL INTERVIEWS, PLEASE LIST YOUR PHONE NUMBER.
OPTIONAL:(   ) _____
      A R E A

THANKS AGAIN.

N O T E S   O N   S O U R C E S

CHAPTER 1

1. "My Generation," Fall 1989 Survey by *Seventeen* magazine, News Corporation of America, New York.

2. Susie Orbach, *Fat Is a Feminist Issue* (New York: Berkley Books, 1978).

3. *Medical Aspects of Human Sexuality*, Spring-Summer 1991.

4. Boston Women's Health Book Collective, *The New Our Bodies, Ourselves* (New York: Touchstone/Simon & Schuster, 1984), p. xvii.

CHAPTER 2

1. Presentation made at the 22nd Annual American Association of Sex Educators, Counselors and Therapists (AASECT) National Conference; by Marty Klein, M.A., M.F.C.C., entitled "Problems of Desire," Crystal Gateway Marriott Hotel, Arlington, Va., February 17, 1990.

2. Shere Hite, *The Hite Report: A Nationwide Study of Female Sexuality* (New York: Dell, 1977) pp. 562–63.

3. Maggie Scarf, *Intimate Partners: Patterns in Love and Marriage* (New York: Ballantine Books, 1987), pp. 257–59.

4. Excerpts from AASECT District One Conference, Omni San Diego Hotel, October 22, 1989; presentation by Sol Gordon, Ph.D.: "Sex Education in the '90s: Politics and Drama."

5. Interview with Faye Wattleton, *Ms.*, October 1989.

CHAPTER 3

1. Karen S. Peterson, "SI Swimsuits Lead Wave of Skin Issues," *USA Today*, February 7, 1990, cover story, Life section, pp. 1–2.

2. Marilyn Elias, "Many Girls Have a Weighty Self-Perception," *USA Today*, 1991.

3. Rick M. Gardner and James A. Morrell, Jr., "Body-Size Judgments and Eye Movements Associated With Looking at Body Regions in Obese and Normal Weight Subjects," *Perceptual and Motor Skills* 73 (1991): 675–82.

4. Susan Brownmiller, *Femininity* (New York: Fawcett Columbine, Ballantine Books, 1985), p. 23.

5. Ibid., p. 158.

6. Alan Prendergast, "Hooked on Perfection," *Special Report on Health*, November 1989, pp. 7–8.

7. Teri Egins, "Forget Hemlines: The Bosomy Look Is Big Fashion News," *Wall Street Journal*, December 2, 1988, p. 1.

8. Elaine Witt, "Image of Beauty," *Chicago Tribune*, Tempo section, February 11, 1990, p. 8.

9. Nora Ephron, "A Few Words About Breasts," *Esquire*, June 1983 (reprint from 1972), p. 324.

10. William Geist, "Star-Crossed Legs," *Egg*, a publication of Forbes, Inc., March 1990, pp. 40–43.

11. William Griffitt and Elaine Hatfield, *Human Sexual Behavior* (Glenview, Ill.: Scott, Foresman & Co., 1985), pp. 360–61.

12. *Psychology of Women Quarterly*, vol. 15 (New York: Cambridge University Press, 1991), pp. 477–88.

CHAPTER 4

1. "Women Being Liberated From Tyranny of Physical Attractiveness as Sole Basis for Their Self-Esteem," University of Maine, Office of Public Affairs, news release, Orono, Maine, October 24, 1991.

2. Mary Ellen Strote, "Mirror, Mirror on the Wall: A Woman Reflects on Sex, Love and Body Image," *Lear's*, June 1991, pp. 35–36.

3. Priscilla Flood, "Body Parts," *Esquire*, June 1981, pp. 35–43; also excerpts from interview with Flood in March 1990, New York City.

4. Gloria Emerson, *Some American Men* (New York: Simon and Schuster, 1985) pp. 235–36.

5. Stephani Cook, "What Do Women Want?" *Gentleman's Quarterly*, October 1987, pp. 280–87.

6. Katharine A. Phillips, M.D., "Body Dysmorphic Disorder: The Distress of Imagined Ugliness," *American Journal of Psychiatry*, September 1991, pp. 1138–47.

CHAPTER 5

1. Melvin Konner, M.D., "Women and Sexuality," *The New York Times Good Health Magazine*, April 29, 1990, p. 26.

2. Kinsey, Alfred C., et al., *Sexual Behavior in the Human Female* (Philadelphia: W. B. Saunders, 1953).

3. Nancy Friday, *Women on Top* (New York: Simon & Schuster, 1991), p. 65.

4. Ibid. p. 273.

5. Esther S. Person, "Some Differences Between Men and Women," *Atlantic Monthly*, March 1988, pp. 71–76.

6. Ibid., p. 74.

7. Jessica Benjamin, *The Bonds of Love: Psychoanalysis, Feminism, and the Problem of Domination* (New York: Pantheon Books, 1988), p. 89.

CHAPTER 6

1. Harriet Goldhor Lerner, Ph.D., *The Dance of Intimacy* (New York: Harper & Row, 1989), p. 3.

2. Maggie Scarf, *Intimate Partners* (New York: Ballantine Books, 1987), p. 47.

3. Lerner, pp. 186–87.

4. Herb Goldberg, Ph.D., *The New Male-Female Relationship* (New York: Signet/Penguin Books, 1983), pp. 25–26.

5. Discussion raised at Barbara DeAngelis seminar, "Say No to Sex and Yes to Love," New York City, sponsor: Learning Annex, held September 1990, Fashion Institute of New York City.

6. Julie M. Rozenzweig, Ph.D., and Dennis M. Dailey, D.S.W., "Dyadic Adjustment/Sexual Satisfaction in Women and Men as a Function of Sex Role Self-Perception," *Journal of Sex and Marital Therapy* 15, no. 1 (Spring 1989): 42ff.

7. John Tierney, "Mind Health," *Vogue*, July 1990, pp. 114ff.

8. Beverly Fehr, "Prototype Analysis of the Concepts of Love and Commitment," *Journal of Personality and Social Psychology* 55, no. 4 (1988): 557–79.

9. Research on sexual behavior outside of marriage presented at press conference on September 5, 1990, by the Kinsey Institute for Research in Sex, Gender, and Reproduction (Indiana University). Supporting information published in *The Kinsey Institute New Report on Sex*, by June M. Reinisch, Ph.D., with Ruth Beasley, M.L.S. (New York: St. Martin's Press, 1990).

10. Scarf, p. 117.

CHAPTER 7

1. Randy Rieland and Sherri Dalphonse, "Sex: The New Rules," *Washingtonian*, February 1992, p. 39.

2. Norman Mailer, *The Prisoner of Sex* (New York: Signet/New American Library, 1971), p. 60.

3. Josephine Lowndes Severly, *Eve's Secrets* (New York: Random House, 1987), pp. 49–139.

4. Boston Women's Health Book Collective, *The New Our Bodies, Ourselves*, (New York: Touchstone/Simon & Schuster, 1984), p. 190.

5. Elizabeth Fenwick and Morris Yaffe, *Sexual Happiness for Women: A Practical Approach* (New York: Henry Holt and Co., 1989), p. 98.

6. June M. Reinisch, Ph.D., *The Kinsey Institute New Report on Sex* (New York: St. Martin's Press, 1990), p. 137.

7. Pearsall, Paul, Ph.D., *Super Marital Sex* (New York: Ivy Books, 1987), pp. 134–35.

8. K. Sookja Chung, Kevin T. McVary, and Kevin E. McKenna, Ph.D., "Sexual Reflexes in Male and Female Rats," *Neuroscience Letters* 94 (1988): 343–48.

9. Dominick Bosco, "Fuel for Love," *Men's Health*, June 1990, pp. 59–61.

CHAPTER 8

1. Felicia Guest, Robert Hatcher, M.D., Felicia Stewart, M.D., and Gary Stewart, M.D., *My Body, My Health: The Concerned Woman's Guide to Gynecology* (New York: John Wiley & Sons, Inc., 1979), pp. 13–15.

2. Boston Women's Health Book Collective, *The New Our Bodies, Ourselves* (New York: Simon & Schuster, 1984).

3. Sally Squires, "Balancing Between Behavior and Biology," *Washington Post*, October 10, 1989, p. 11.

4. Jamie Talan, "Hormone Flunks PMS Test," *New York Newsday*, July 18, 1990, p. 6; Peter J. Schmidt, et al., "Lack of Effect of Induced Menses on Symptoms in Women With Premenstrual Syndrome," *New England Journal of Medicine* 324, no. 17, April 25 (1991): 1174–79.

5. Interview with Gail Brockman, M.D., Los Angeles, CA, December 1989.

6. Mary Jane Gray, M.D., Florence Haseltine, M.D., et al., *The Woman's Guide to Good Health*, Yonkers, N.Y.: Consumer Reports Books, 1991.

7. Phyllis A. Guze, M.D., "Pelvic Inflammatory Disease (PID)," *Health Insights* newsletter, University of California, Los Angeles, September 1989, pp. 1, 5.

8. Felicia Guest, et al. *My Body, My Health*, p. 525.

9. Jimmy M. Sparks, M.D., "Vaginitis," *Journal of Reproductive Medicine*, 36, no. 10 (October 1991): 745–51.

10. Niels Lauersen, M.D., "Update on Contraception," *Cosmopolitan*, November 1988, p. 271.

11. Barbara Donlon, "Softening the 'C' Word," *Boston Herald*, April 30, 1989, p. 1.

12. David Noonan, "Special Deliveries," *Special Report: on Health*, May–July 1989, p. 44.

13. DRUGS/ALCOHOL section: American Psychiatric Assn./National Women's Health Network, update on percent mood-altering, legal drugs prescribed to women vs. men . . . (update Jan. 1992).

14. Gina Kolata, "N.I.H. Neglects Women, Study Says," *The New York Times*, June 19, 1990, p. C6.

15. Bruce Lambert, "AIDS in Black Women Seen as Leading Killer," *The New York Times*, July 11, 1990, p. B3 (report on Centers for Disease Control study published in *JAMA*).

16. Interview with Robert Rolfs, Ph.D., researcher and spokesman for federal Centers for Disease Control, Atlanta, July 1990; Robert Byrd, "U.S. AIDS cases top 200,000 mark," *Boston Globe*, January 17, 1992.

17. Michael R. Kagay, "Poll Finds AIDS Causes Single People to Alter Behavior," *The New York Times*, June 18, 1991, p. C3.

18. "AIDS Medicines in Development: Drugs and Vaccines," Pharmaceutical Manufacturers Association, Washington, D.C., Winter 1990.

19. Miriam Stoppard, M.D., *Everywoman's Medical Handbook* (New York: Ballantine Books, 1989), p. 123.

20. Interview with Margaret Webb, American Social Health Association, Research Triangle Park, NC, 1992.

21. Boston Women's Health Book Collective, *The New Our Bodies, Ourselves* (New York: Touchstone/Simon & Schuster, 1984), p. 273.

CHAPTER 9

1. Effectiveness rates of contraceptives discussed and confirmed in interviews with Planned Parenthood personnel in Chicago and Phoenix; representatives of the Alan Guttmacher Institute in New York City; Dr. Robert Hatcher, professor of obstetrics and gynecology at Emory University in Atlanta; Dr. Albert George Thomas, assistant professor of obstetrics and gynecology, Mt. Sinai Medical Center, New York City, and statistics published in Felicia Guest, Robert Hatcher, M.D., Felicia Stewart, M.D., and Gary Stewart, M.D., *My Body, My Health: The Concerned Woman's Guide to Gynecology* (New York: John Wiley & Sons, Inc., 1979).

2. James Thornton, "Adherence of Adherents," *Corporate Report Minnesota*, January 1987, pp. 39–44.

3. Barbara Brotman, "Study Urged on Birth Control," *Chicago Tribune*, January 29, 1990. Sec II, p. 1, 4.

4. "Cervical Cap Compares Well to Condom and Diaphragm," *The Washington Post*, October 10, 1989, Health, p. 22.

5. *AMA Journal*; various authors, April 12–15, 1989; *Newsday* report, "Two IUDs Called Safe"; April 18, 1989).

6. *The Lancet*, Summer 1990 issue, 2-page opinion on long-term use of IUDs.

7. Sara Davidson, "Dr. Rock's Magic Pill," *Esquire*, December 1983, p. 100.

8. Mark Baker, "Men on Abortion," *Esquire*, March 1990, pp. 120, 122.

CHAPTER 10

1. Stephen L. Corson, M.D., *Conquering Infertility: A Guide for Couples* (New York: Prentice-Hall, 1991), p. 6; Dorling Kindersley Limited and the AMA, *The American Medical Association Encyclopedia of Medicine* (New York: Random House, 1989), p. 586.

2. Interviews with obstetrics-gynecology staff at Mount Sinai School of Medicine; Mount Sinai Medical Center, New York City, spring and summer 1990.

3. The Boston Women's Health Book Collective, *The New Our Bodies, Ourselves* (New York: Touchstone/Simon & Schuster, 1984), p. 342.

4. Corson, p. 1.

5. John Newton, FRCOG, and Dr. Dorothy Tachhi, "Long-term Use of Copper Intrauterine Devices," *Lancet* 335 (June 2, 1990), 1322–23.

6. Sheila Kitzinger, *The Complete Book of Pregnancy and Childbirth* (New York: Alfred A. Knopf, 1982), p. 328.

7. Information from lectures and discussions in Prepared Childbirth classes, Mount Sinai Medical Center, New York City, summer–fall 1990; instructor, Johanna Gordon, R.N.

8. Beverly Savage and Diana Simkin, *Preparation for Birth: The Complete Guide to the Lamaze Method* (New York: Ballantine Books, 1987), p. 217.

9. Jane E. Brody, "Personal Health: As Breast-feeding Is More Widely Accepted in U.S., Recent Studies Shatter Myths," *The New York Times*, August 10, 1989, p. B10.

10. Elisabeth Bing, "Yes, You Can," *Childbirth*, vol. 7, no. 2 (Newton, Mass.: Reed Publishing/Cahners Publishing Co., 1990), pp. 29–30.

11. Savage and Simkin, p. 343.

12. David Laskin, "Sex and the New Father," *American Baby*, June 1989, pp. 41–43.

BIBLIOGRAPHY

Baulieu, Etienne-Emile and Mort Rosenblum. *The "Abortion Pill."* New York: Simon & Schuster, 1991.

Benjamin, Jessica. *The Bonds of Love: Psychoanalysis, Feminism, and the Problem of Domination.* New York: Pantheon, 1988.

Bohannan, Paul, ed. *Divorce and After.* New York: Anchor Books/Doubleday, 1971.

Camp, John. *Plastic Surgery: The Kindest Cut.* New York: Henry Holt and Co., 1989.

Castleman, Michael. *Sexual Solutions.* New York: Touchstone/Simon & Schuster, 1980, 1989.

Cousins, Norman. *Head First.* New York: Penguin Books, 1989.

Curtis, Glade B. *Your Pregnancy Week-by-Week.* Tucson, AZ: Fisher Books, 1989.

Cutler, Winifred and Celso-Ramon Garcia. *Menopause.* New York: W. W. Norton, 1991.

Emerson, Gloria. *Some American Men.* New York: Simon & Schuster, 1985.

Ford, Clellan S. and Frank A. Beach. *Patterns of Sexual Behaviour.* London: Eyre & Spottiswoode, 1952, 1965.

Freedman, Rita. *Bodylove.* New York: Harper & Row, 1988.

Friday, Nancy. *Women on Top.* New York: Simon & Schuster, 1991.

Friedan, Betty. *The Feminine Mystique:* Twentieth Anniversary Edition. New York: Norton, 1983.

Goldberg, Herb. *The New Male-Female Relationship.* New York: Signet/Penguin Books, 1984.

————. *What Men Really Want.* New York: Signet/New American Library, 1991.

Gray, Henry. *Gray's Anatomy.* New York: Bounty Books/Crown Publishers, 1977.

Guest, Felicia, Foberth Hatcher, Felicia Stewart, and Gary Stewart. *My Body, My Health: The Concerned Woman's Guide to Gynecology.* New York: John Wiley & Sons, 1979.

Henig, Robin Marantz. *How a Woman Ages.* New York: Ballantine Books, 1985.

Hite, Shere. *The Hite Report: A Nationwide Study of Female Sexuality.* New York: Dell, 1977.

Institute for Advanced Study of Human Sexuality. *The Complete Guide to Safer Sex.* Fort Lee, NJ: Barricade Books, 1987, 1992.

Jastrow, Joseph. *Freud: His Dream and Sex Theories.* New York: Permabooks/Greenberg, 1959.

Jennings, Chris. *Understanding and Preventing AIDS.* Cambridge, MA: Health Alert Press, 1992.

Keen, Sam. *Fire in the Belly.* New York: Bantam Books, 1992.

Kitzinger, Sheila. *The Complete Book of Pregnancy and Childbirth.* New York: Alfred A. Knopf, 1982.

Knopf, Jennifer, Michael Seiler, and Susan Melstsner. *ISD: Inhibited Sexual Desire.* New York: William Morrow and Co., Inc., 1990.

Mailer, Norman. *The Prisoner of Sex.* New York: Signet/New American Library, 1971.

Malesky, Gale and Charles B. Inlander. *Take this Book to the Gynecologist with You: A Consumer's Guide to Women's Health.* Reading, MA: Addison-Wesley, 1991.

Masters, William H., Virginia E. Johnson, and Robert C. Kolodny. *Crisis: Heterosexual Behavior in the Age of AIDS*. New York: Grove Press, 1988.

Mayer, Nancy. *The Male Mid-Life Crisis: Fresh Starts After 40*. New York: Signet/New American Library, 1979.

Morgenstern, Michael, Steven Naifeh, and Gregory White Smith. *How to Make Love to a Woman*. New York: Clarkson N. Potter, 1982.

Norris, Ronald V. and Colleen Sullivan. *PMS: Premenstrual Syndrome*. New York: Rawson Associates, 1983.

Offit, Avodah K. *The Sexual Self*. New York: Congdon & Weed, Inc., 1983.

Orbach, Susie. *Fat Is a Feminist Issue*. New York: Berkley/Paddington Press, 1978.

Pearsall, Paul. *Super Marital Sex*. New York: Ivy Books, 1987.

Penney, Alexandra. *How to Keep Your Man Monogamous*. New York: Bantam Books, 1989.

Pesmen, Curtis. *How a Man Ages*. New York: Ballantine Books, 1984.

Reinisch, June M. and Ruth Beasley. *The Kinsey Institute New Report on Sex*. New York: St. Martin's Press, 1990.

Rosenfield, A., M. F. Fathalla, A. Germain, and C. L. Indriso. *International Journal of Gynecology & Obstetrics: Women's Health in the Third World: The Impact of Unwanted Pregnancy (Supplement 3)*. Limerick, Ireland: Elsevier Scientific Publishers, Ireland, Ltd., 1989.

Rubin, Lillian B. *Erotic Wars: What Happened to the Sexual Revolution?* New York: Farrar, Straus & Giroux, 1990.

Savage, Beverly and Diana Simkin. *Preparation for Birth: The Complete Guide to the Lamaze Method*. New York: Ballantine Books, 1987.

Scarf, Maggie. *Intimate Partners: Patterns in Love and Marriage*. New York: Random House, 1987; Ballantine Books, 1988.

Shapiro, Howard I. *The New Birth Control Book*. Englewood Cliffs, NJ: Prentice-Hall, 1988.

Spitzer, Robert L., Andrew E. Skodol, Miriam Gibbon, and Janet B. W. Williams. *A Psychiatrist's Casebook (The DSM-III Casebook)*. New York: Warner Books, 1981.

Steinem, Gloria. *Revolution from Within: A Book of Self-Esteem*. Boston: Little, Brown & Co., 1992.

Stone, Robert L. *Essays on the Closing of the American Mind*. Chicago: Chicago Review Press, 1989.

Stoppard, Miriam. *Everywoman's Medical Handbook*. New York: Ballantine Books, 1988.

Tannen, Deborah. *You Just Don't Understand*. New York: Ballantine Books, 1990.

The Boston Women's Health Book Collective. *The New Our Bodies, Ourselves*. New York: Touchstone/Simon & Schuster, 1984.

Thompson, D. S., ed. *Every Woman's Health: The Complete Guide to Body and Mind by 15 Women Doctors*. Englewood Cliffs, NJ: Prentice-Hall, 1985.

Westheimer, Ruth. *Dr. Ruth's Guide to Good Sex*. New York: Warner Books, 1983.

Wilson, Josleen. *Woman: Your Body, Your Health*. New York: Harvest; Orlando, FL: Harcourt Brace Jovanovich, 1990.

Yaffe, Maurice and Elizabeth Fenwick. *Sexual Happiness for Women: A Practical Approach*. New York: Henry Holt and Co., 1988.